HOPE

February 2018

HOPE
MAGAZINE
*"Supporting the
Brain Injury Community"*

HOPE MAGAZINE

Serving All Impacted by Brain Injury

February 2018

Publisher
David A. Grant

Editor
Sarah Grant

Contributing Writers
Tobie-Lynn Andrade
Virginia Cote
Kelly Davis
David A. Grant
Tris Greenman
Norma Myers
Amy Northridge
Drew Palavage

*FREE subscriptions at
www.TBIHopeMagazine.com*

Welcome to the February 2018 issue of HOPE Magazine!

I would like to personally extend a warm welcome to all our new readers. Next month we will celebrate the three-year anniversary of our magazine – and what an amazing three years it has been.

Since the launch of HOPE Magazine back in March of 2015, we have quickly grown to become the largest publication worldwide serving the brain injury community. We have thousands of readers worldwide. It's humbling to envision a reader in Nepal finding hope as someone in Ghana or Kenya finds the same end of isolation.

This month's issue features a blend of writers old and new, with voices familiar to regular readers mixed with several brand new contributors.

While we cannot take away the fact that brain injury may be part of your life today, it is our heartfelt hope that we can make your journey just a bit easier.

Peace,

David A. Grant
Publisher

Contents

"The word 'happy' would lose its meaning if it were not balanced by sadness."

~Carl Jung

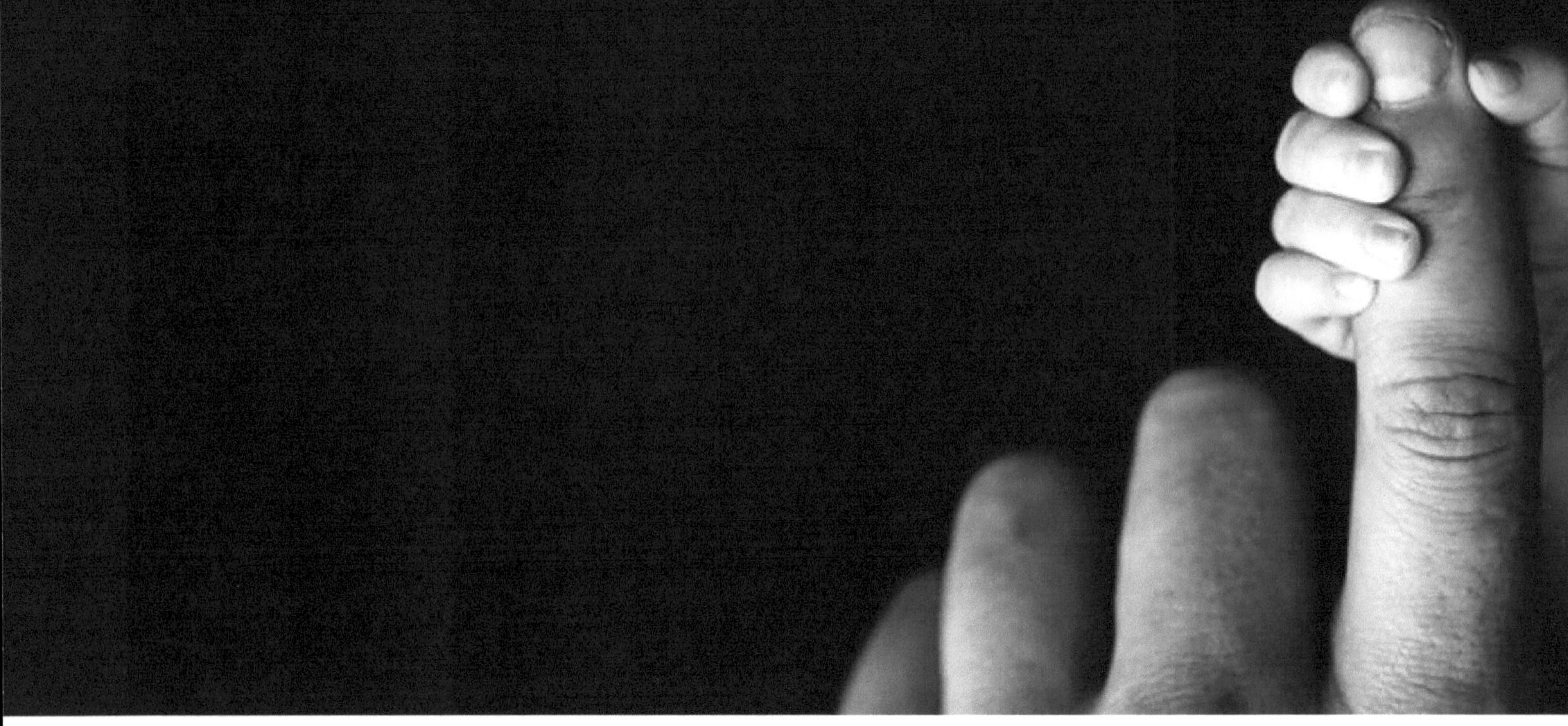

Parenting After Brain Injury
By Kelly Davis

Living with a brain injury can often feel like trying to navigate one of those large corn mazes. You feel that things are going well until you hit a dead end. Then you start to re-evaluate where you stand in life and every decision that has lead you to that point.

Living with a brain injury and parenting young children can feel like you are navigating the maze with a blindfold on, with someone strapped to your legs, someone asking you the same question repeatedly, and you just touched something sticky where sticky shouldn't be. Over the past four years of my own journey with a brain injury, I have learned these five lessons.

> "Living with a brain injury and parenting young children can feel like you are navigating the maze with a blindfold on."

Have a support system

My family would not have survived the first two months after my injury without my mother and mother-in-law taking turns being available 24/7. They prepared all the meals, took care of my kids, and did all the housekeeping. Even now, I still could not survive without them. They still help with driving the kids to/from school and watching them on days when I am not doing so well.

Having a support system is crucial - it does not have to be family. There are many avenues for support including friends or possibly your local religious group. Let your friends know what you are going through. Name some specific troubles/difficulties you may be having. They may offer to bake a meal or take the kids for an afternoon. Admittedly, I did not take advantage of this.

There are also local brain injury support groups that may work for you later in your injury journey. It's wonderful to have a group of people who understand exactly what you are feeling, either symptom-wise or emotionally. I highly recommend connecting with a group whether it is online, or in person.

Have a retreat plan
You are going to need a plan for retreat. There are going to be times when you absolutely need a brain break for 20-30 minutes. These are the times when you feel like you might splinter into a million pieces.

This is when I use technology to my advantage. Most of the time I will put on a movie for the kids. Despite their age differences, I can usually pick a movie that will keep everyone engaged. Sometimes, I split them up with 1-2 kids downstairs and 1-2 kids upstairs for separate movie times. Then I can lie down in my quiet bedroom or use strategies from my "toolkit" that work for me to relax and regroup.

It is vital to keep a written copy of the toolkit. This is a list of your tried and true methods to bring relief.

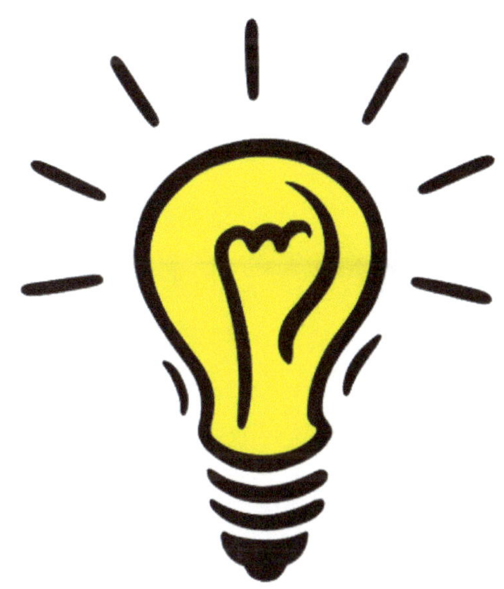

"I use technology to my advantage. Most of the time I will put on a movie for the kids. Despite their age differences, I can usually pick a movie that will keep everyone engaged."

I suggest writing it down because when you are in a brain breakdown it's hard to think of or remember what works for you.

Examples of what's inside my toolkit include: a heating pad, ice packs, Sea-Bands, essential oils, meditation suggestions, deep breathing, slow walking, ear plugs, and getting some fresh air.

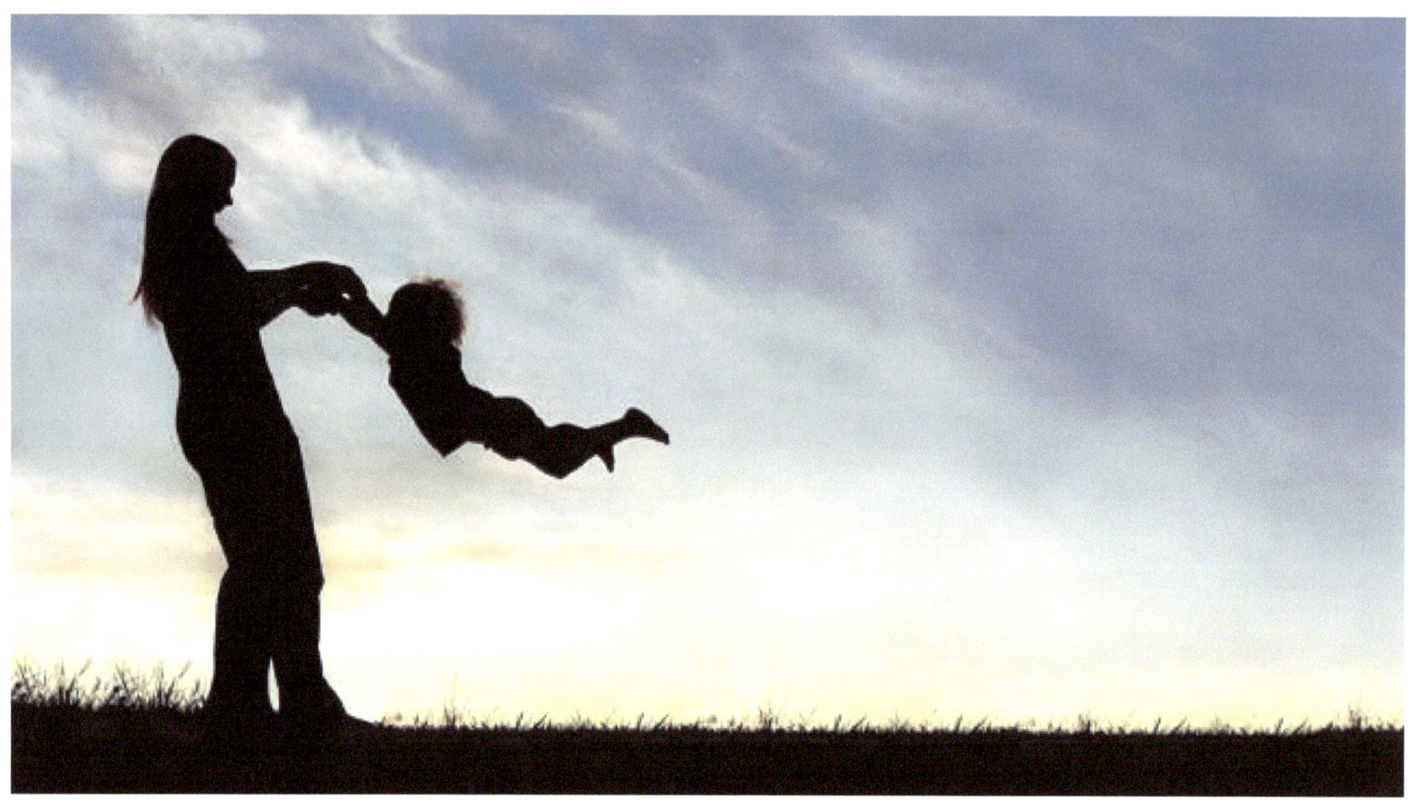

Letting go of perfection

I believe Disney's Elsa said it best while belting out her song that is forever imprinted on parents' brains: *"Let It Go!"* As parents, we may be self-judging about how we are doing, what we are feeding our kids, or how clean our house is. It's in these moments that we need to give ourselves grace. One of my biggest challenges was accepting that I was going to have down days.

Instead of trying to fight it and swim upstream, which usually made it worse, I learned to let myself rest and regroup. I let myself give the kids cereal or fruit and yogurt for dinner. I know that letting go of the need to cook a full meal was helping me in that day to heal, and most likely I would be back at it tomorrow. The world wasn't going to end, if today I sat on the couch with my eyes closed and I didn't get to cleaning the bathrooms or folding the laundry. That could all wait until the next day or later.

My life changed when I finally learned and started to follow this simple strategy. I was able to let go of the parental guilt, or the "I should be," and truly let myself heal and rest when I needed to. Once you are able to embrace this you can feel yourself begin to relax and reduce stress.

Know your limits and stick to them

Knowing your limits is directly related to the last lesson of letting go. We all, at some point, wish for our former self or want to be back to our "normal." Being aware that I will not get back to Kelly 1.0, but being able to make Kelly 2.0 be the best version, is something that I can work on. I know that I can't get up early with the kids, make breakfasts, put in laundry, work, go to school functions, and meet up with friends. So why do I try and then get upset and frustrated when I dig myself into a hole trying to do it all? Being able to say no to others and yourself, is a skill to be learned.

I know that getting up in the morning is the worst time for me. My kids bursting with energy and the chaos of the morning is too much for my sensitive brain to handle. What I am able to do is to help my oldest son before the younger two get up. With the lights dimmed and the relative quiet of the downstairs I can assist in the morning routine. Once the other two kids come into the picture, my husband is ready to take over and I retreat to the quiet bedroom for about 30 minutes. Knowing that how I address the morning sets up how I will respond to the rest of the day helps me to set my limits and stick to them.

Enjoy your loves
Last, but not least, is to enjoy your family. My injury happened when my kids were five years, two years, and nine-months old. So much of those first couple of years I spent shushing them or spending limited time with them. But it's so true that time goes by fast, and they are only little once. Now I cherish every moment with them. By using the first four lessons, I am able to be a bigger part of my family and my children's future.

My hope is that these words help you in some way, and that you believe you can and that you will have a fulfilling life with your children and family.

Meet Kelly Davis

Kelly Davis is a mother of three very active boys, a physical therapist, and a brain injury survivor. She never imagined that having a fall in her own home could change her life so much. She feels very lucky to have a wonderful and supportive family, including her husband of ten years.

She would love to use her own experiences to help others in the brain injury community and hopes to reach more people with her new writing career. Currently her biggest dream is to adopt a yellow Labrador retriever and name him Pudding.

You can read more about Kelly and her injury and other writings on her website www.quiet-storm.blog.

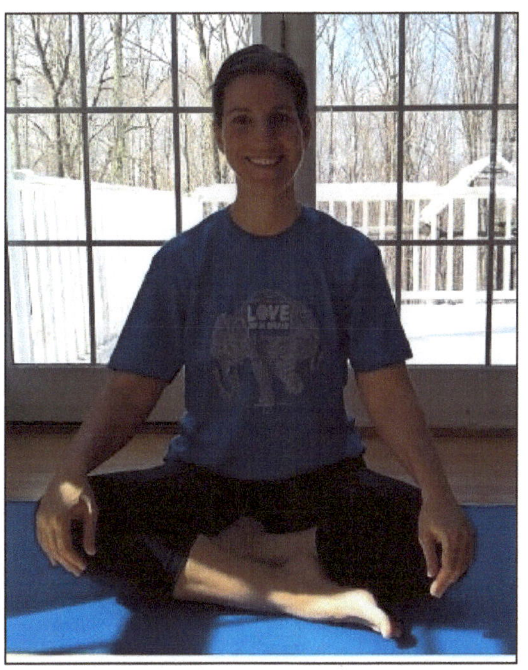

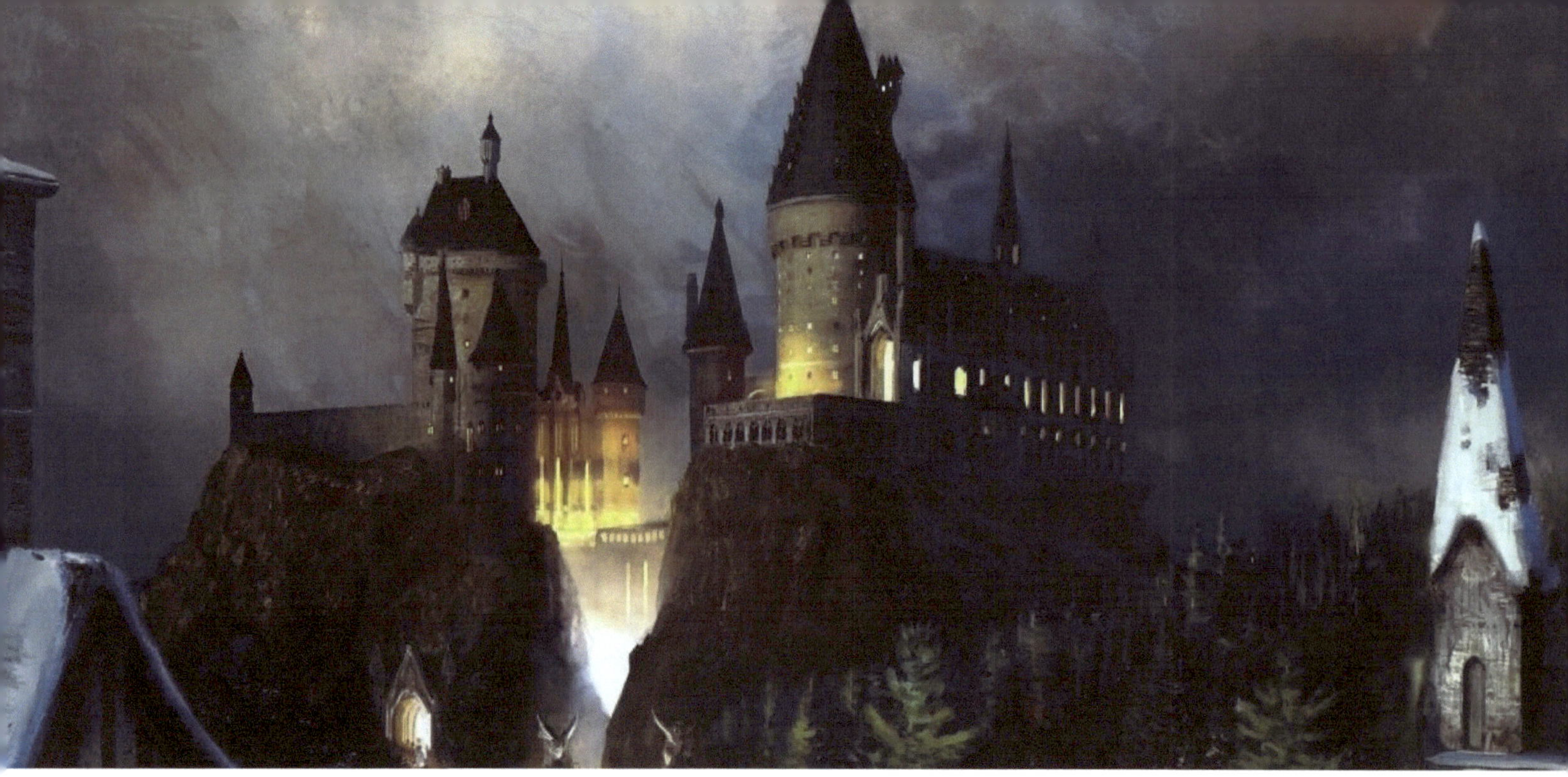

My Invisibility Cloak

By Tobie-Lynn Andrade

Anyone who knows me will attest that I am a huge Harry Potter geek and can relate just about anything to the experiences of "The boy who lived." The concept of an invisibility cloak seems pretty cool: tuck yourself under its folds and you can explore to your heart's content, observe and interact, without being seen. Before my injury I could fantasize about what I could do with a cloak of my own, and then I realized I was wearing one permanently.

> "I have always been outspoken and tact has never been my strong suit."

I have always been outspoken and tact has never been my strong suit. I have used my words and my voice to share, heal, hurt, educate, soothe, inform, argue, love and hate. I know the nuances of volume of speech, rhythm and timing. I am well read, and can use words big and small. Despite all my past experiences with words, and the fact that I am still speaking aloud, I am no longer heard.

I have become invisible in many ways.

I was a successful business woman, both for a well-established craft company and a partner in my husband's health clinic. I was balanced between both worlds by attending trade shows, designing patterns, selling crafts at local shows and making herbal salves and lotions for the clinic. I was equally competent and comfortable in both worlds. I no longer work, have acquaintances, or the energy or desire

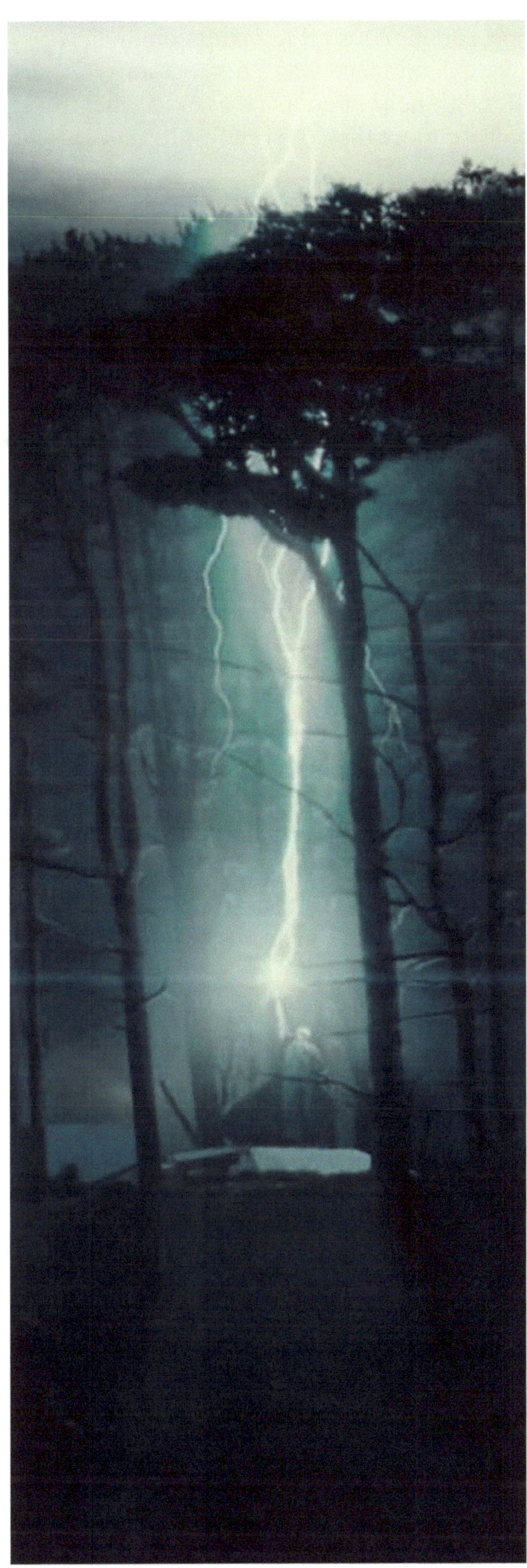

to create. I lost all but one "friend" from my previous work life, not to mention my income, my purpose, my joy for crafting. My work identity and my independence were gone.

Even my private pleasures became difficult; aphasia made it hard to communicate what I wanted or needed. Reading was no longer the escape it used to be - having to look up the meanings of words, write reminders on post-it notes about which characters were married to who, to follow the story line. I couldn't concentrate on knitting patterns, or enjoy hours with wool and clicking needles any longer. My identity as a crafter was gone.

Family life even became a struggle as roles were changed. Suddenly, I was the one needing a caregiver, having someone clean and cook for me and drive me around, took even more away. My husband and parents had to step in and make sure someone was with me all the time to care for me during and after seizures, to take care of our pets when I was too weak or fatigued to do it myself. I became a drain on their time and energy. My husband lost several jobs after he closed his clinic to take care of me. I became his patient. He took care of my medication and therapy schedule and my mother became our support, chauffeur, cook, housekeeper, and nurse when he was at work. My role within my family was gone.

I didn't become invisible immediately following my injury. I did try to work part time, but was unable to continue my job. Co-workers invited me to cookie exchanges and social gatherings, but it was very uncomfortable having seizures or not fitting into the conversation any longer.

I recall a conversation about the number of dozens of cookies we needed to make at the exchange, and I said I was quite proud of myself that I was able to go to the store (with Mom) and budget and buy the ingredients for my contribution (baked with Mom), and was met with that awkward silence I have become all too familiar with.

I had said something unusual, something that no one could relate to. How could they know what a triumph it was for me to have planned a recipe, budgeted for it, shopped for, and baked? I won't even mention how hard it was to actually sit in a group of people who used to be my peers and focus all my attention on the conversation and not stuttering or acting confused. That awkward admittance was a descent into invisibility as far as my work relationships were concerned. It didn't help of course that even when we had Facebook, I was often unable to sit at or look at a computer for more than the briefest of times... and thus my online invisibility began as well.

Even at home, I was becoming slowly less and less visible. The dog would go to my husband or parents for snacks and her outdoor time; meals were planned and made without my input; the house was cleaned in an order that wasn't mine, and my beloved books and knitting projects sat neglected while I tried to make sense of life after brain injury.

During my seizures, I had brief moments between actual seizures where I wasn't quite lucid or vocal, but I could hear just fine. It's like hearing your nurse and doctor talk just outside the room about your diagnosis when they don't think you can hear. It was the same with family and friends.

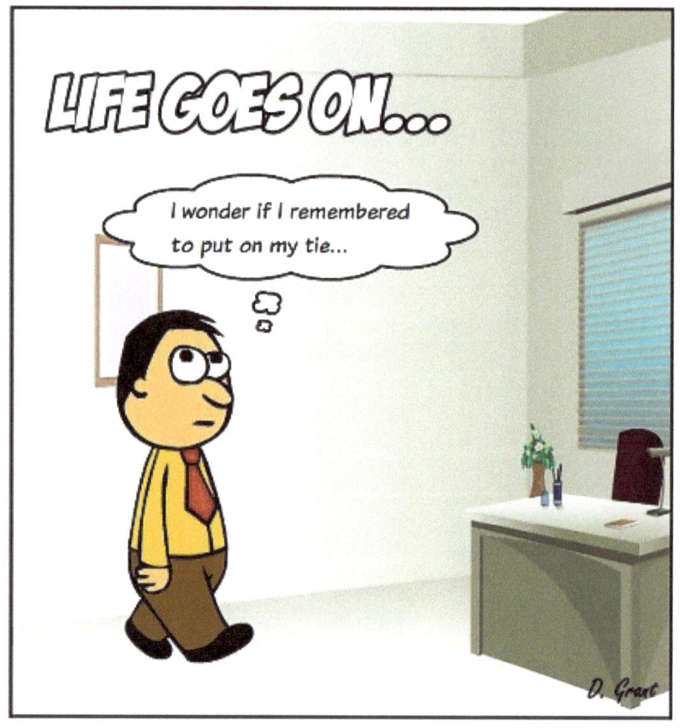

I recall someone who didn't visit often, nor understand my seizures, comment in one of those non-lucid moments that I would be better off left in a nursing home or hospital where my family wouldn't have to see or take care of me. It's probably best that I couldn't comment at that time. My words would have had quite the bite. I did notice that my family didn't respond. Invisibility at home was almost complete.

Doctors' visits and hospital stays are their own trials with a brain injury. I have seen a huge variety of medical staff, and their manner goes from respectful to rude and every place in between. Only a very minute percentage of them actually aim questions at me, ask my input, or talk directly to me like I am part of the conversation (let alone the reason for being there).

Many ask questions over my head to my husband or mother who accompanied me for so many visits, despite my being in the room. I even recall a few very rude ones who would ask my husband or family questions and then "shush" me when I tried to answer. I have even been told that as a person with a brain injury I wouldn't understand what they were asking and told I could sit in the waiting room if I couldn't be quiet. I've been told that recovery ends after one year post injury, and other half and full untruths. I've been told all the things I will not ever do again, and to just give up on trying to be something I never will be again. Some of those things I heard the medical professionals tell my family, as if I wasn't in the room listening and understanding the words. I was invisible in the doctor's office.

Being bombarded with questions and not having the time to respond is just as hard as not being listened to. I was partially paralyzed following a seizure and the doctor was throwing fast questions at me:

"Can you feel this?" (touching my knee)
"Do you understand what I am asking you?"
"Can you feel this?" (touching my ankle)
"Can you speak?"
"Can you feel this?" (touching my toe)"

I was so overwhelmed that by the time I was able to answer the first question with a NO and the second with a YES we were both having two very different conversations. I was invisible in the examination room.

Experiences like the one with the doctor are sadly all too common with a brain injured patient. But the results of such communication lapses (Invisibility) are quite harmful. Just last fall I was taken by ambulance to the hospital when my husband was unable to control my seizures. After hours in the emergency room and all the drama and overstimulation that occurs there, I told the nurse I was thinking of killing myself.

I told the doctor as well, and my family was there at that point. I asked for help, said I was depressed and unable to cope with my life anymore, I didn't want to live and that if they sent me home I would find a way to kill myself. My family stepped up and told the staff that I was fine, just overtired, that I wasn't a risk to myself, that it was just my brain injury talking. I actually punched my husband in the face repeatedly in the hospital, something I had never ever done before and was totally out of character for me.

I told the staff again not to let me go home, that I would kill myself. They listened to my family, wrote up the report that I was unable to make decisions for myself, and sent me home. I was invisible in the emergency room.

Clearly I didn't kill myself when I went home, but only because I was only so angry at how insignificant and invisible I had become that I was determined to change it.

I went home and threw myself into crafts and things that were previously enjoyable. I worked hard at making a Harry Potter Christmas Tree topped with the Sorting Hat and other themed holiday decorations. I made sure Christmas was special. The kids each got personalized photo albums filled with memories, hand-knitted gifts for family, and a visit with the few people I count as friends. A friend who knew me before my injury was talking to one who met me post-injury about my tree, filled with my own handmade ornaments. The newer friend commented how much I am able to do, even with a head injury, while the older friend responded "you should have seen what she could do before." I wasn't meant to overhear that comment and pretended I didn't. It hurt me quite deeply for a while, and then I took stock of how it was said, not maliciously at all, kind of wistfully. I realized then that the old me, the before-my-injury me is invisible. Still remembered, but no longer here.

To again refer to the novels, Harry Potter starts off life not knowing he's famous, destined to battle one of the most evil powerful wizards of all time. He uses his strengths, relies on his wit, learns how to overcome the darkness, and for the most part does it all without wearing his cloak of invisibility. I've decided I'm due for some magic of my own and am shedding my cloak of invisibility too. My injury may be invisible, but I will not be. This will be my year to be heard, even if it started as an angry whisper only I could hear, telling me to live.

I am doing more of what I enjoy, taking joy in little things, celebrating my achievements and milestones. I am trying to take better care of myself, listening to my cues and symptoms and limitations. I am still pushing for improvements with my memory and energy levels and acceptance. I am getting treatment for myself. I am learning to accept who I am now. I am trying to find my identity, my independence, my new role in my family. I am in therapy to banish the suicidal thoughts. I will struggle, but eventually I will talk and people will hear me and see me again, and whoever I am, I will no longer be invisible.

Meet Tobie-Lynn Andrade

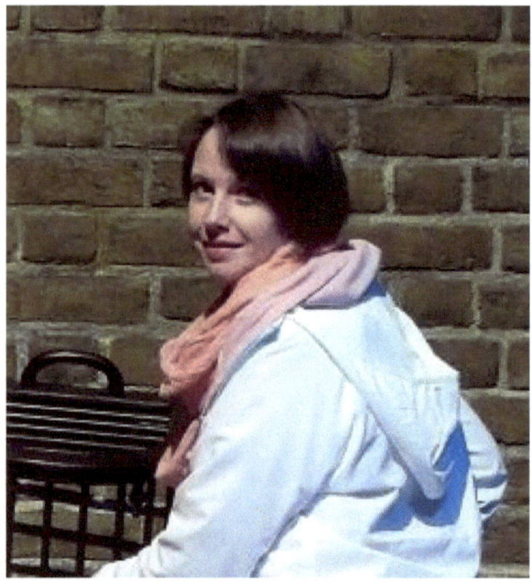

Tobie-Lynn is a lifelong fan of reading and an avid crafter, as well as a huge Harry Potter geek. She is recovering from a grade three concussion with front left lobe damage and post-concussion syndrome with seizures.

Tobie-Lynn is using natural medicines and methods to heal from her injuries, and the Harry Potter stories to help herself heal. One of her greatest moments in life was going to England where the Harry Potter series was filmed and standing with her husband on the actual bridge used in the films.

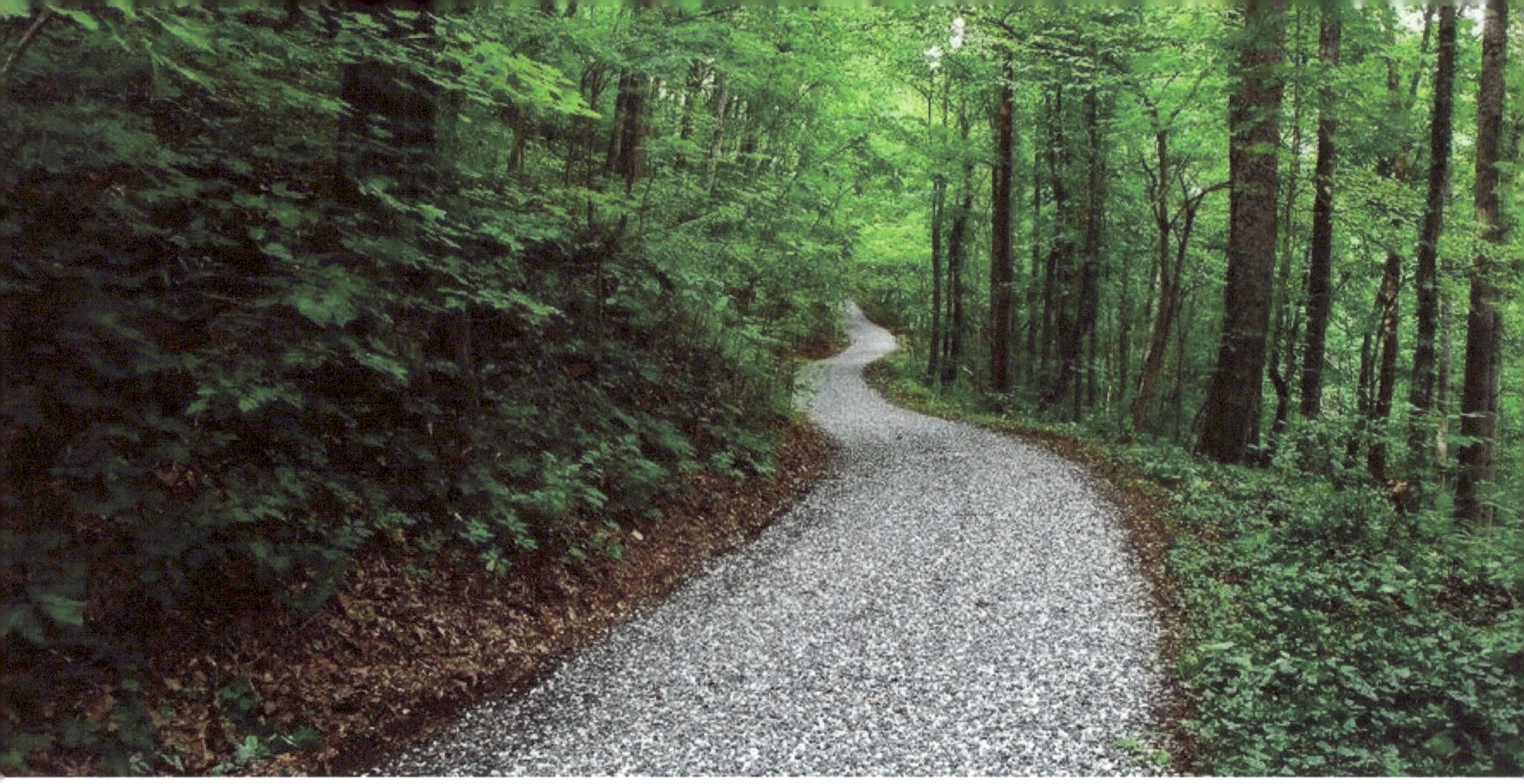

Guardian from the Universe

By Tris Greenman

One of our grandsons proclaimed he was "Guardian *of* the Universe," the other day while playing with his brothers. I began thinking of myself as a guardian *from* the universe. My husband's June 2013 accident left him with a traumatic brain injury. After two months in a coma, another in acute care getting off the ventilator and a stint in a rehabilitation hospital, I found myself in the role of guardian. I barely remember sitting in the courtroom and being appointed his legal guardian. I brought him home from rehab even though he still did not know who I was or where he lived.

Guardians are appointed for individuals who are deemed by the court to be mentally disabled or incapacitated. It was a quick process for us, as Tim's condition was critical. He did not have durable power of attorney or medical directives in place prior to the accident. The doctor signed a form; I was interviewed by a court appointed guardian ad litem who then recommended the guardianship to the court. Done. There is something about the legality of it that added weight to the already overwhelming situation we were in. I was Tim's guardian. I was responsible for his medical decisions along with financial ones.

> "Guardians are appointed for individuals who are deemed by the court to be mentally disabled or incapacitated."

If you are familiar with my life before Tim's accident, you know that Tim and I were anti-drama. We live in the middle of the woods, opting out of the suburban hubbub. When you turn into our long driveway, calm descends and it truly is a special place.

After Tim's accident, I became involved in the whole legal issue of settlement negotiations. Everyone assumed that since the driver of the utility truck was cited for running the stop sign, Tim would be getting a large settlement. He did not. Out of the woodwork came the ne'er-do-wells that prey upon the disabled.

Brain injury survivors often have difficulty with judgment. They can be spontaneous and irrational. Two days after Tim was home, so-called friends (and relatives) visited asking for money, vehicles, tools and equipment. Tim did not even remember who some of these people were.

He was overwhelmed, to say the least, but it was I who had to step in and say no. Suddenly I was not only trying to figure out how to live with Tim's brain injury but this added dilemma of greed. I wanted to shut everyone out.

Early on, he had no memory of the daily therapists coming in and spending time with him, but his generous nature shone through as he demonstrated his regard for someone by trying to give them something from our home.

He had no attachment to anything sentimentally, so if you liked a picture or a chair, he offered it to you. "You want this?" "Let me give you something." The therapists educated me on impulsivity as one of the effects of a TBI, as well as politely refusing Tim's offer of gifts.

Tim's generosity didn't stop with just therapists. We were inundated by family and friends after his homecoming, and amazingly, a number of them took the things he offered. I was

> "Early on, he had no memory of the daily therapists coming in and spending time with him, but his generous nature shone through as he demonstrated his regard for someone by trying to give them something from our home."

dumbfounded. I ended up standing in the middle of our driveway blocking a so-called friend from driving off on one of Tim's vintage bikes.

Time after time I found myself saying no to both Tim and his intended recipient, often becoming the bad guy. I don't want this to be a negative article, I really would like to help educate those affected by TBI - both patients and caregivers. It doesn't have to be a battle, I just had to learn and adjust.

Set limits. Tim has his own little space in the heated garage where he receives friends and visitors. It is set up with a stereo, coffee pot, small fridge and snacks. There is no need for anyone to come into the house, thus eliminating our personal items from being given away or reviewed. Tim has shelves of trinkets in his space. He loads these with items he has painted, made, found or purchased. He knows he can give anything away on these shelves without "asking permission." It doesn't hamper his generosity and makes him feel good.

In turn, I have re-examined the value of things in our life and let go of a lot of items. Life's really not about things. Identify and hide the truly precious ones that have been handed down or hold a special place in your heart. Some articles can never be replaced and we don't need to lose any more pieces of ourselves than we already have.

> "Block phone calls from solicitors - some tend to prey upon the elderly and disabled."

There is a limit on withdrawals on his bank account and I get text alerts when money is taken. At the end of the day, we write down what he spent in a journal so he can see the effect of spending money. This makes him more conscientious of the value of money, basically re-training him in the finances of life. Once again, I find myself a little more generous with charities, family and friends, hoping that giving a little more will help someone as I myself have been helped in the past few years.

Block phone calls from solicitors - some tend to prey upon the elderly and disabled. Block channels with infomercials from the TV. Go through the mail, tossing out the mass of requests for money, but pick one or two to discuss with your family so that you can decide together if and how much, and then track the donations. Reviewing the money going out routinely has been a big help when discussing with Tim his desire to hand out a twenty here and there to visitors.

As his guardian, I was expected to make medical decisions about recommended therapies and medications. Of course I did what the doctors suggested, but continually questioned whether or not I was doing the right thing for Tim. It was a lot of pressure balancing out what I wanted to happen with what I knew Tim would want. I didn't think so at the time, but shortly before Tim's accident he had a good friend who suffered from a stroke and passed away. After watching his friend's family care for him for five long weeks, Tim voiced his opinion on what he would want should such an event occur with him. I was thankful for this conversation, as it gave me guidance for making medical decisions for Tim, we just didn't have the paperwork drawn up.

I encourage everyone to have these discussions with family members now. Get medical directives in place, communicate your own wishes. If you are a caretaker, it is that much more crucial to write down or let someone know your directives for medical care. Create a detailed notebook on the doctors, therapists, aides, finances, likes and dislikes of your injured loved one along with unique tricks that have helped you care for him/her.

Being prepared has been the best defense in navigating the new world of brain injury. We need to share our experiences with each other to help spread the awareness and let each other know we are not alone in this universe.

Meet Tris Greenman

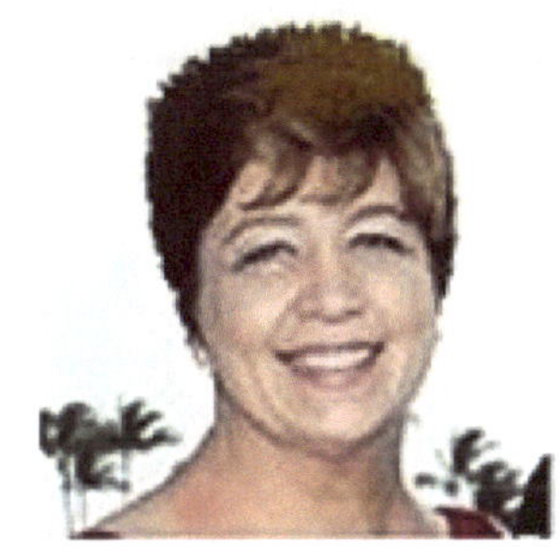

Tris Greenman is caregiver to her husband Tim in Southwest Michigan. She manages a full-time job in addition to partnering with Tim to manage his brain injury. They enjoy the outdoors, grandkids and nightly games of cribbage. "Caregivers Unite!"

Editor's Note: With Tris' recent submission, came a short note. It read, in part, *"Four days after writing this article, my husband Tim was involved in a tragic accident at home and passed away. He was an amazing person. I am sure his brain injury played a role."* Our hearts and prayers go out to Tris and her family, and to those who lost their struggle with post-injury life.

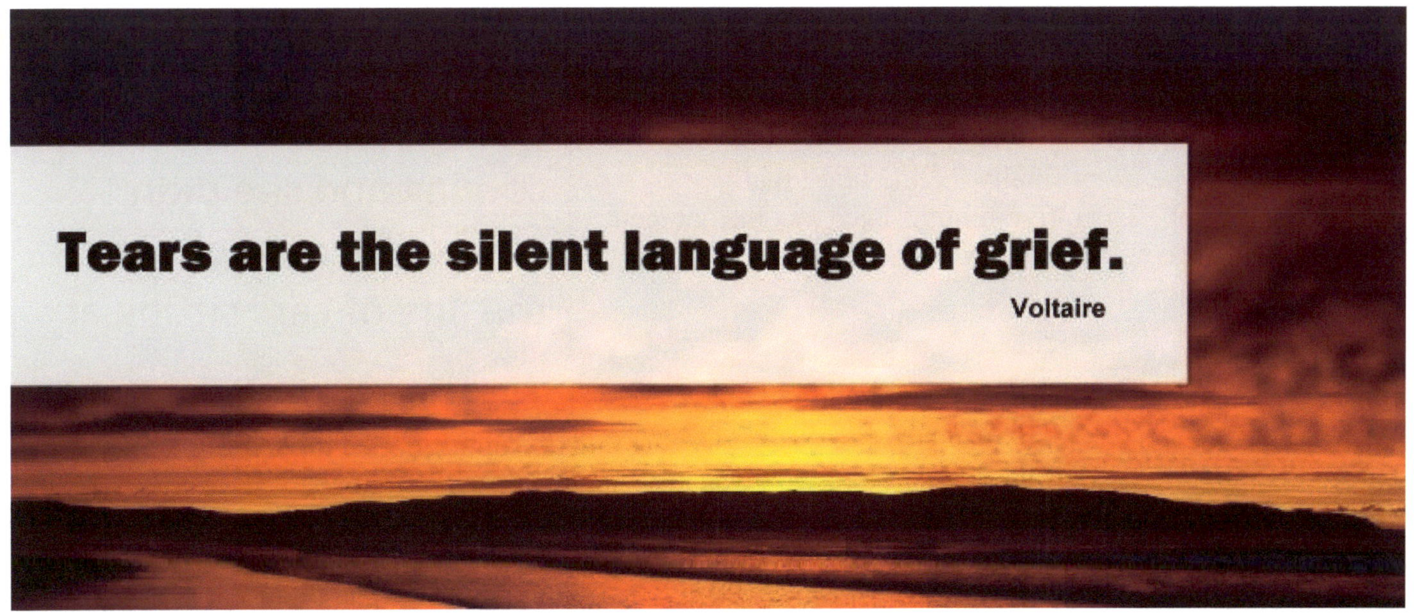

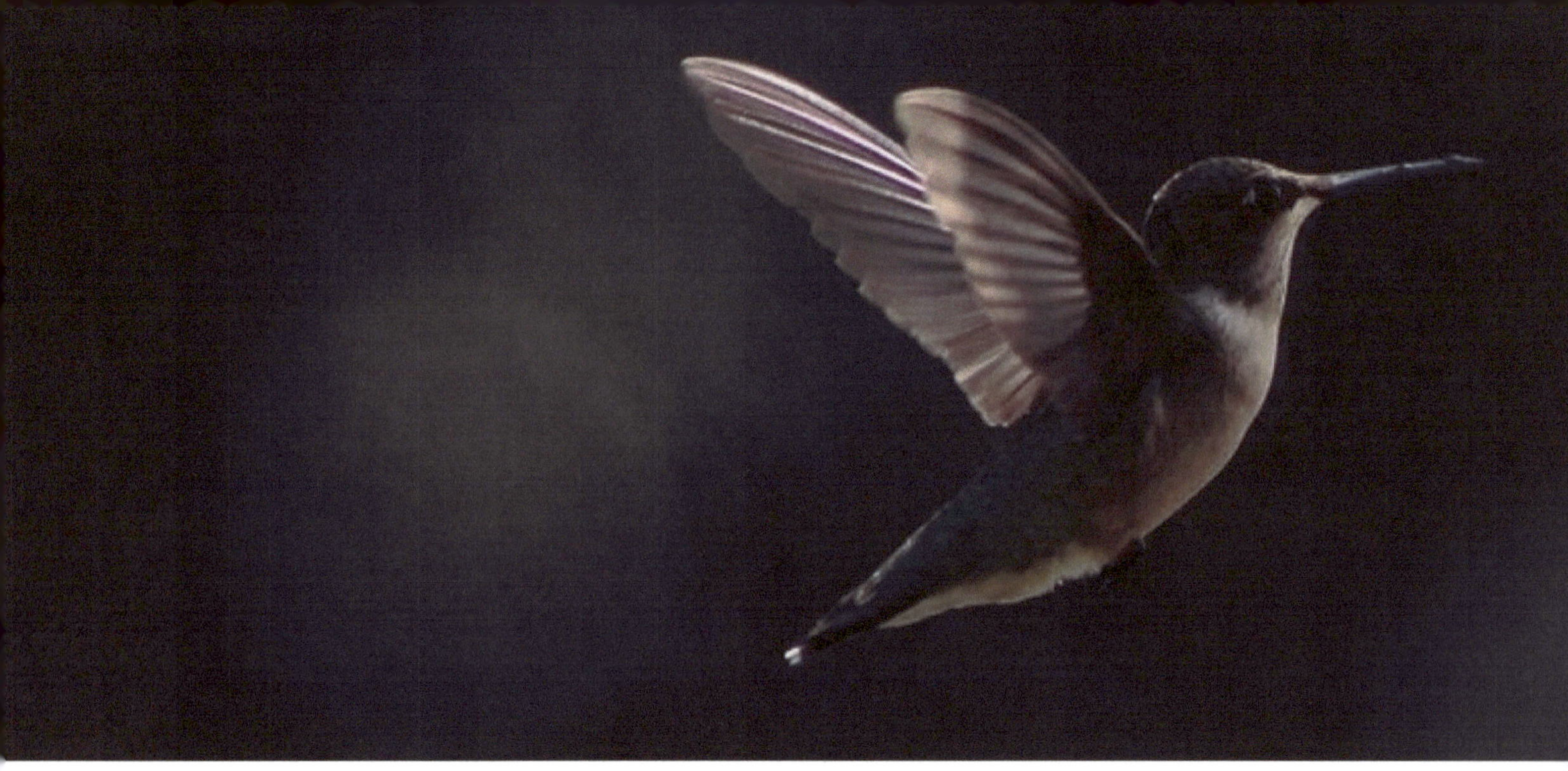

Who Are You?

By Amy Northridge

Alice in Wonderland has always been one of my favorite books and now that I don't really read, it's a tale I retell to myself at night when I fall asleep. 'Who are you?' asks the Cheshire Cat so innocently— and the question in and of itself sends Alice into a panicked state.

On my 30th birthday, I remember having a sense of peace. Not the peace of a life well-lived and knowing all of the answers, but the peace of finally feeling like I really understood myself. Then, five-months later was the accident. I was sitting in the middle row of our SUV with my then two-year-old son.

We were sitting at a red light. We were silly dancing to Sesame Street ABC's, and then I think I heard a noise.

> "We didn't see the car coming and she didn't notice the red light or the line of cars sitting at it."

That's all I really remember. We didn't see the car coming and she didn't notice the red light or the line of cars sitting at it. Thankfully my husband, who was driving, had left plenty of space between us and the car in front of us. I remember that I immediately reached for my son—it took me months and two specialists for someone to ask if I really remembered the accident. I don't think I do, but who can really say?

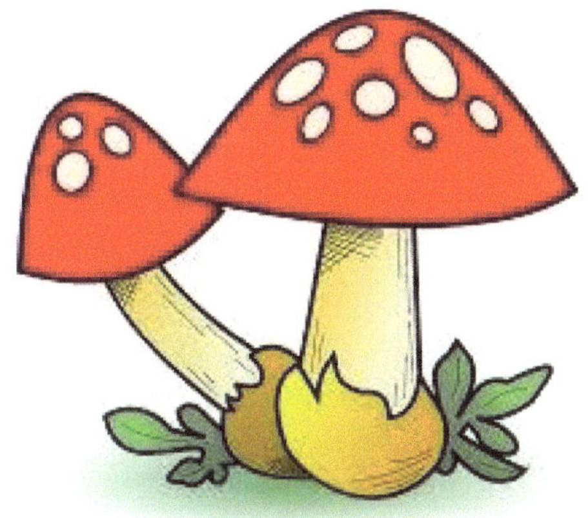

It was sometime last summer, nearing the year post-injury mark, when doctors started talking to me about my new normal. If you're reading this, I'm sure you know what I'm talking about. It's a moment you brace yourself for, if you've been in the support groups and done all of the reading. I'd nearly completed two types of post-accident therapy and I thought I'd run out of new things to tell my neurologist, besides the fact that everything has stayed basically the same with slight improvements, and so I was waiting for "the moment." The moment when you feel the people in the room who you need to fight to help make you better, settle on the fact that from now on you'll just be different. And maybe someday you'll forget what your old normal was, which I imagine is challenging when you have trouble making new memories. Who are you? And once you figure it out, will you remember?

Soon after that appointment, my family was at our local summer church camp serving as chaplains and the heavens opened up--the rains fell. And camp was quiet. My husband was out trying to rescue hikers from the downpour and my son slept. So I sat on the porch and waited for life to start again. There I sat, camera in hand. Watching the rain drops. Waiting for answers.

And then, the hummingbirds started coming. They came over and over again for food at the feeder in front of me. I settled in and I watched them. I felt joy in the midst of confusion. And frankly, I mainly remember this moment because I took an absurd amount of pictures of it. The hummingbirds, the flowers, the raindrops—all memories of the healing power of water for the soul. I don't know who the new normal me is, but the new me loved this moment.

When I got home from camp, I changed my profile picture on Facebook to one of my hummingbird shots, proud to have gotten some nice pictures. (Well, they were nice pictures after I edited them to account for the fact that my vision is off so all of my pictures taken in the midst of fatigue start crooked.) I was feeling joyful to have a good profile picture that isn't of this woman I don't really understand or recognize as myself. And it was that day something changed for me. I don't know if you can call it hope, but it certainly isn't acceptance of the "new normal," or understanding of who I am today. But, it was something. Something that day shifted inside of me and I knew that I'd be different still the next morning when I awoke.

You see, a friend of mine who works with young children with disabilities commented on my new profile picture. She wasn't meaning to be profound or to change my life. It was just a simple comment that she loves hummingbirds. They make her think of her students working so hard to stay in the same place. I saw this and forgot to breathe for a moment. That's me! I'm a hummingbird now. And all of a sudden I felt there was beauty in the struggle I'm going through. There's beauty in living a life in gratitude for good moments and simple pleasures. There's beauty in working hard to stay in one place.

Somedays now I think about getting a hummingbird tattoo near the site of the injury. Something the "me who existed before the accident" never would have done, but that the new me desires because I want some mark to show that I'm changed. I'm not sure I'll ever make that jump. But what I do know is that whether it is permanently on my skin or not—I'm beautiful in this moment—even if I'm directing all my energy into staying in place and learning the new me - and you are too. So, keep holding on when you are feeling lost like Alice, and know that your struggle, your fight, your triumph in the moment – big or small—is beautiful, just like you.

Meet Amy Northridge

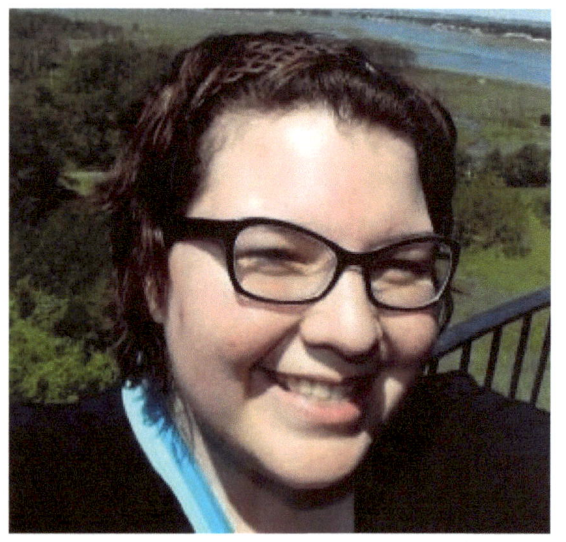

Amy is currently working her way out of the tunnel of the internal struggles following a not so mild, mTBI. Amy works as a pastor in the Evangelical Lutheran Church in America and is grateful every day to be surrounded by the most gracious community and supportive colleagues. She is blessed with fantastic parents, siblings, and extended family. She also has a tremendously supportive husband, and a rock star toddler who has learned empathy and care in ways that will never stop amazing her.

Courage is resistance to fear, mastery of fear, not absence of fear.

~ Mark Twain

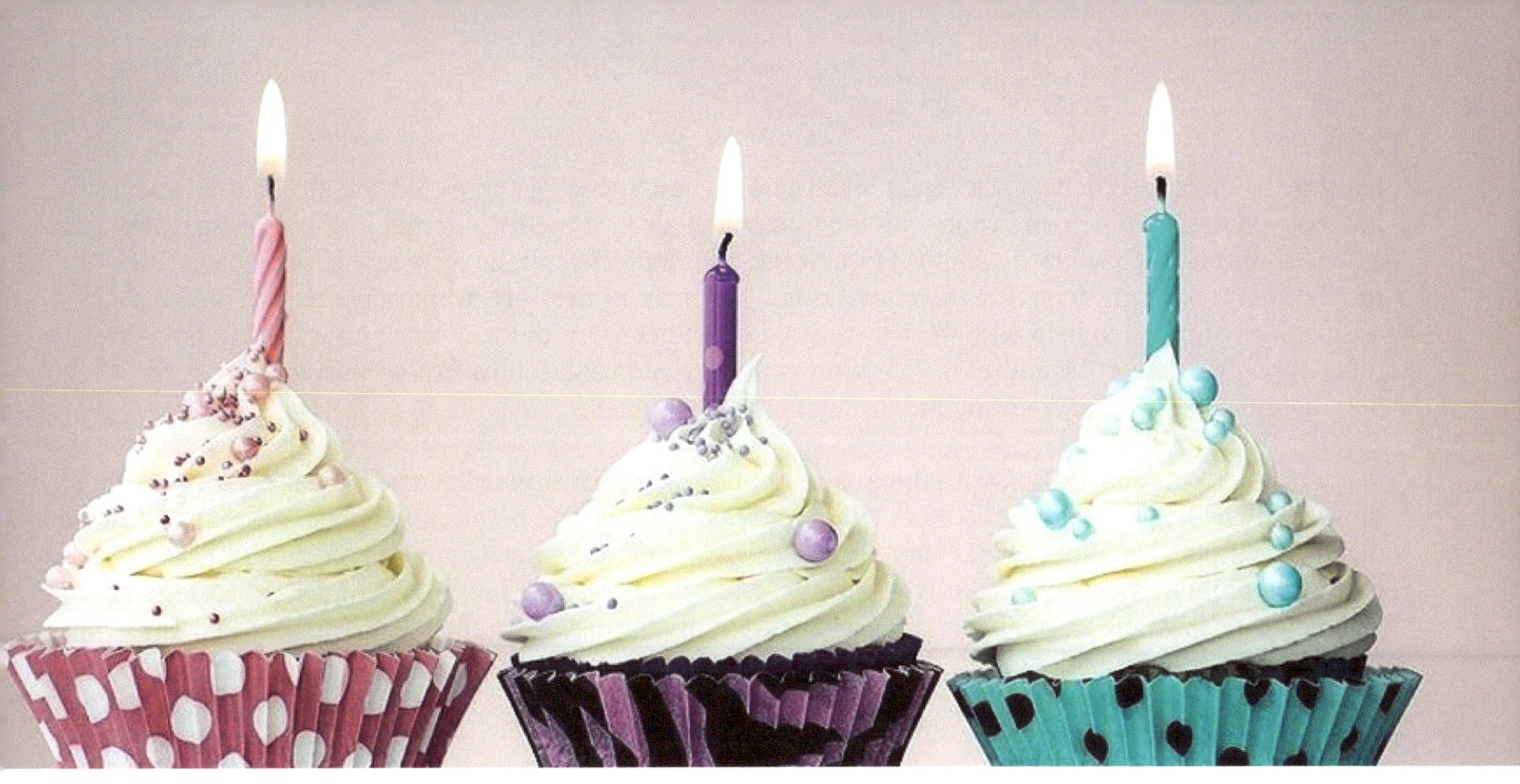

Three Years Out
By Drew Palavage

It has been almost three years since my snowboarding accident that resulted in my brain injury and about two years since my first submission to HOPE magazine. I thought a breakdown of what has helped me, what has been "therapeutically neutral," and what has been detrimental might help others new to brain injury as well as what has been cathartic to me.

I was in a snowboarding accident in Vermont back in March of 2015. I suffered a *DAI (diffuse axonal injury)*, as well as a couple of other things, with the DAI/TBI being the most long-term/life-changing. I was very "physical" before the accident and was engaged in a lot of sports and physical pursuits. I did work in a Neuro-ICU so I knew everything that was going on with me.

> "Almost three years later, I have realized that cognitively I am all there."

Almost three years later, I have realized that cognitively I am all there. My wife and others would agree. I do not even get headaches any longer, but physically I still have challenges. I am still wobbly on my feet and have balance issues. I am weak on the right side with neuro pain/pins and needles in the arm and leg. I continue to be dysarthric, which means I sound like I am drunk, but it is slowly improving. I have a constant ringing in my ears, and I still have double vision though it has been corrected a bit with surgery and prism glasses.

I still go to Physical Therapy, Occupational Therapy, and Speech Therapy. I have also started seeing a neuropsychologist to help me cope with the loss and change of the former me. I have a history of minor concussions and was worried about CTE (chronic traumatic encephalopathy), which is what a few football players get from having their "bell rung" too many times. My primary doctor put me on a low dose anti-depressant to help with the low times. I don't get suicidal ideation anymore. I still have low times though. I am very thankful for a loving family, friends and fellow brain injury survivors for helping me cope with, and getting me through the rough times.

What has been hard is dealing with the loss of the physical self. How I have been dealing with this is I do as much as I can. I work out at least every other day. I alternate between weights, paddle and rowing machine, elliptical, stationary bike and a treadmill. This not only makes me feel physically better but perhaps more importantly – mentally. I push myself relatively hard. I also do as much around the house as I can. This is where an understanding wife and family has been a godsend. This includes taking out the garbage and recyclables, raking leaves, snow blowing, cooking/grilling and general home maintenance.

These things make me feel useful and glad to be alive. I've also been out on a kayak (I used to race outrigger canoe competitively), been on a three-wheeled bike (I'm in the process of re-learning a two wheeler) and - drum roll please - I've got my official driver's license back! I do use a spinner knob and a left foot accelerator as legal modifications. I can drive better than I can walk.

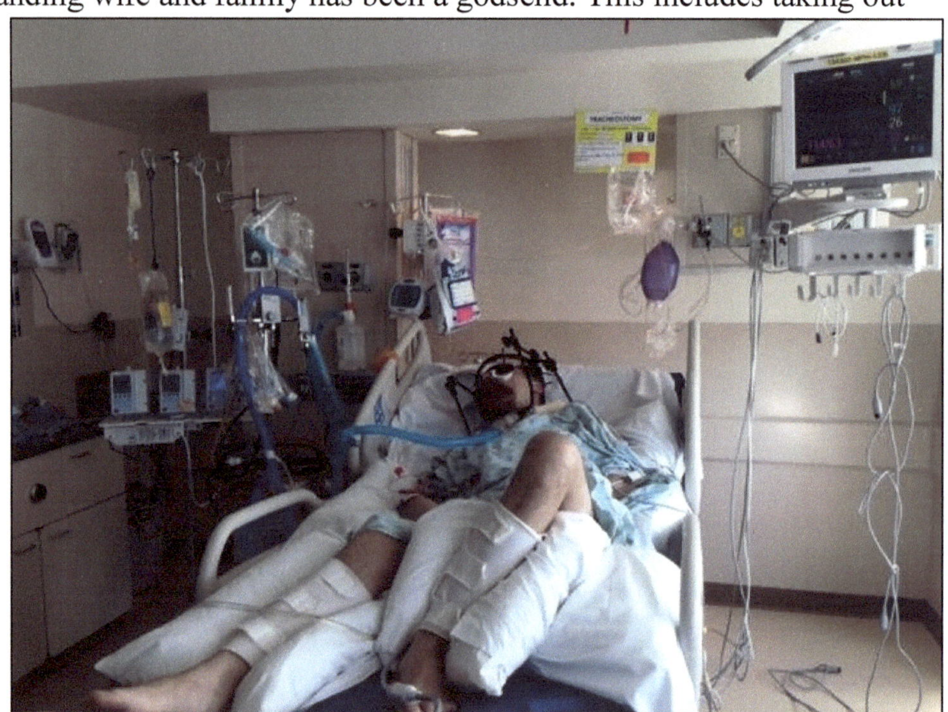

Drew after his Accident

Another thing that has been very helpful is the companionship of a good pet. In my case, a dog, Kia. He accepts and wants to be around me always. He does not care if I do not walk fast or that I speak with a slur. Taking him for a walk in the woods every morning has been good therapy for me (walking on unstable ground) and getting outdoors. I am not sure who benefits more, him or me.

I have achieved some lofty goals over the last couple of years and my future goals are to:

1) Join the gym at rehab and work out with others allowing more socialization
2) Ride a two wheeled bike "comfortably"
3) Stay in relatively good shape
4) Paddle my one-person outrigger canoe that I used to race
5) Learn to tread or keep my head above water (I used to swim like a fish. Now I sink like a rock)
6) Continue to get better with my balance and speech

7) Take a trip on a plane (my wife eventually wants to take a river cruise)
8) Continue to go places (out to eat, store, etc.)

I want to stay active. After a brain injury, you should try to play an instrument, engage with others, push yourself, and try things! I believe this helps to re-map the brain. For example, I am amazed with how much I can do now as a "lefty."

Things that are not so good for me are:

Idle time. For me, sitting around all day watching TV is not good. I feel lousy and unmotivated. I try to get outside a bit every day, even if it's a -20 degrees wind chill outside. My doctor agrees.

Blaming others. I have found that in general, people want to be helpful. If they are too helpful, just kindly let them know. Try to be a bit humorous and a pleasure to be around. Sure, you might not get as much pity but folks will like to be around you. I never questioned "why me?" I rather like to look at it like this: how many times have we said or read that when someone's child is sick or in an accident, people say, "Why couldn't it be me?" I used to love to snowboard with my daughter. I am 100% grateful that this happened to me and not her. That is how I like to look at it. I still get really down in the dumps now and then but doing some of the above things and lessening the others seems to definitely help. I may not be where I want to be, but at three years out I am better than I thought possible!

Meet Drew Palavage

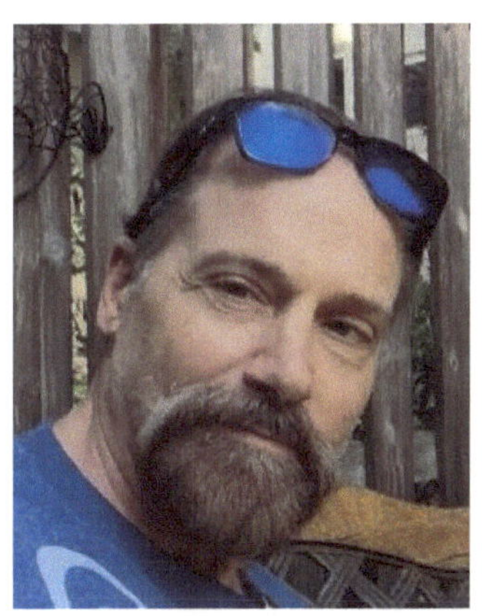

Drew takes pride in being a good husband and father. He was/is also a fierce competitor and will work hard every day.

He enjoys working out and maintaining his home. Very much a goal-setter, he is looking forward to future gains as his brain injury recovery continues.

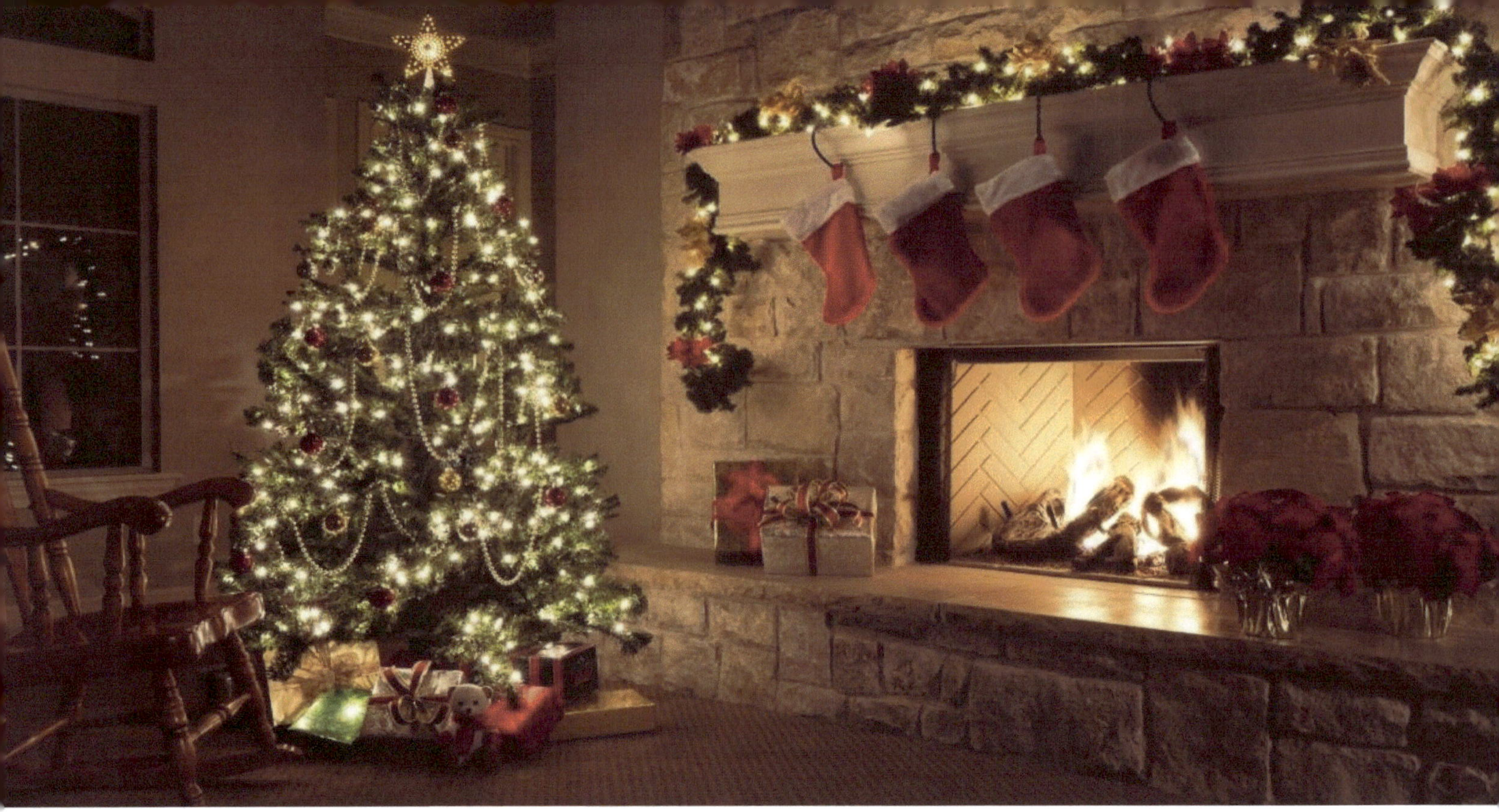

A Geocaching Christmas

By Virginia Cote

My son Rod had been looking for a hobby, one that would challenge his brain and help in his recovery from a brain injury. He discovered Geocaching. Geocaching uses coordinates on a GPS device to find hidden items, or caches.

These caches are hidden all over the world and they come in all different sizes and all different levels of imaginations. In the past four months he has found 149 caches. He had not dreamt in the beginning that he would be anywhere near finding so many. He also had not dreamt that he could claim a "First Time Find." FTF's means you are the first person to find a newly planted cache and he has found nine so far. This is quite an accomplishment for someone who has to push his brain so much harder just to get through the day. Another challenge for Rod is also due to his injury he has lost a lot of his eyesight, making his finds harder and longer than most. He has walked miles and miles to find these caches, not just so he can add his name to a small piece of paper and record his find, but so he can know inside himself that he has worth.

This year for Christmas, I decided to add some geocaching presents. His stocking included things like tweezers and flashlights. I also shopped at the geocache site adding a "Lego box" to his pile of gifts. I found an Ammo box at a grain store that I filled with items one might find in a cache, all individually wrapped and placed inside. What turned out to be his best present was a medium size box that his wife, Marlyn wrapped by first taping a tiny little cache to the bottom and then filled the box with different kinds of packing such as; Styrofoam peanuts, shopping bags, tissue paper and old, already popped bubble wrap. I had found a micro waterproof container in the hardware store designed for boaters to keep a pill safe and dry.

It was small and it had another, even smaller, container inside. It was the smaller container that Marlyn taped inside the box. Inside this tiny container I put a tiny note that said, "The Cache is in the tree." Inside the larger part of the cache was a $100 dollar bill, folded over twice the long way and tightly rolled and mashed inside. This one I hung on the tree.

I love my Christmas tree and I love every ornament I put on it. Each year, I try to get Rod to look at my beautiful tree and each year he looks but doesn't really see, as he says, "nice job mom." So this year when he read the note, "The cache is in the tree" he was excited to look for it. He soon discovered that it wasn't like looking in a tree out in the woods. This tree was full of all kinds of sparkly things.

He quickly scanned up and down the tree and knew right off this would take some time to find. After five minutes he began to laugh as he said, "You have found a way to make me really look at your tree." He had to look at each and every ornament.

He looked high and low, deep inside and on the outer tips, going over and over each and every inch of the tree. Then he began to think as I would, "No, mom is short she wouldn't put it up high. Would she hide it close to the trunk or is there an ornament she could hide it inside."

Finally, he scrunched down real low to the floor and bent around to the back of the tree and there it was in plain sight. A big grin came onto his face and he began to laugh. It had taken a half hour or so to find. He then had to use his new tweezers to get the money out from this newest found cache, but the money was not the highlight of the gift; when geocaching it is always about the find. My reward was a great big hug.

Meet Virginia Cote

Virginia writes…

"I have been helping my son, Rod Stokes with his recovery from a brain injury. It has been a big learning process for me. He is the one that hunts and finds ways to challenge his brain. I support and encourage him and I am his transportation. "

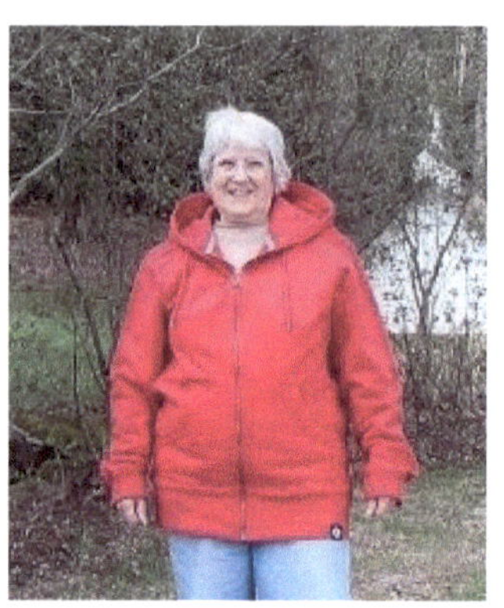

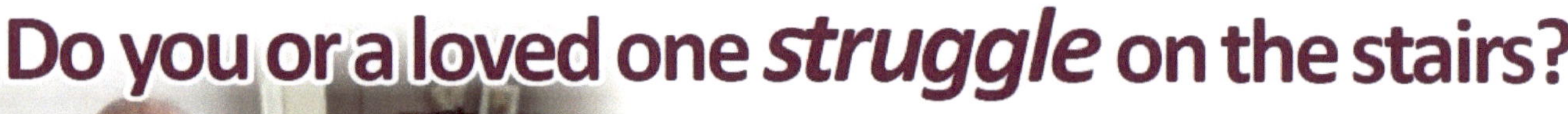

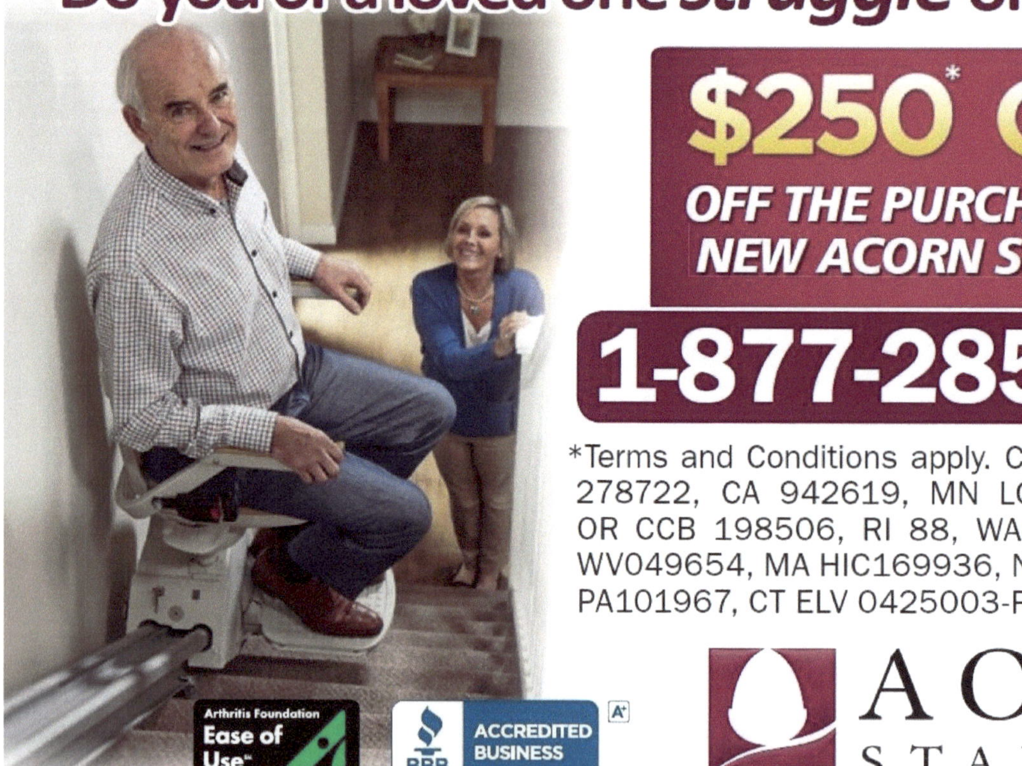

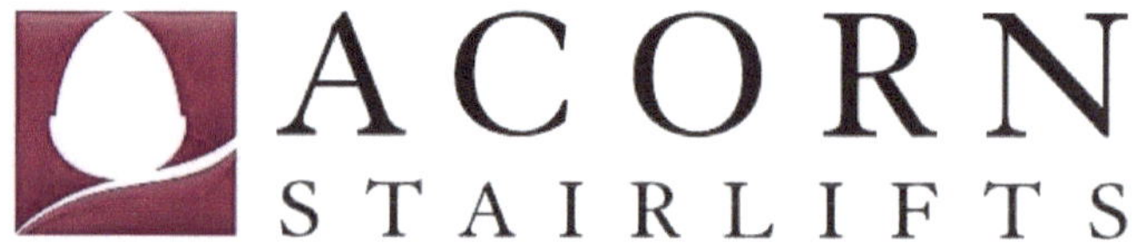

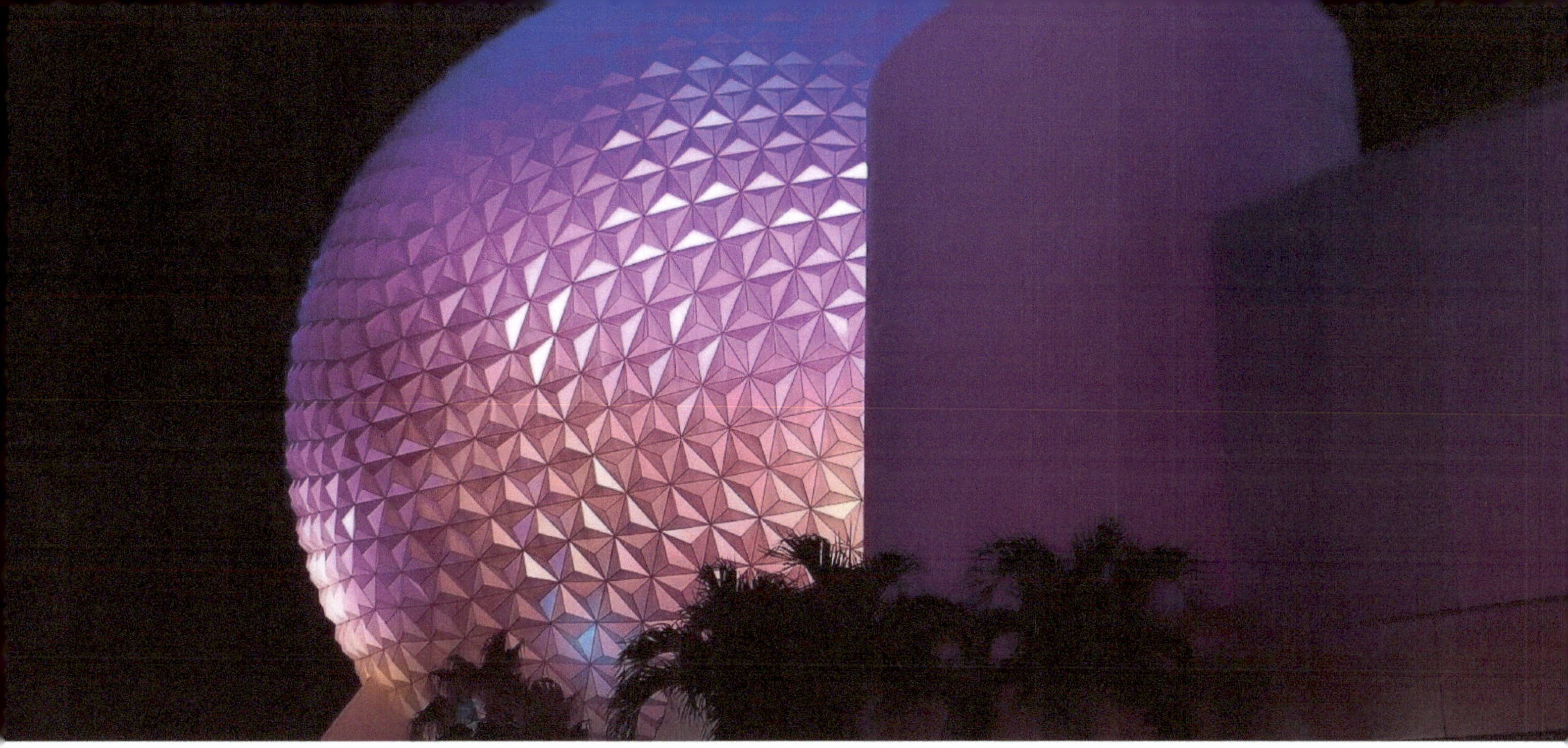

The Magic of Disney
By David A. Grant

Many years ago, I learned that there is something special that happens when a couple of brain injury survivors are together. We "get" each other. You can tell me many things about yourself – if you are part Irish, we have a commonality. If you happen to be a fellow New Englander, we share a geographic common denominator. If you are a firstborn child, we can share that experience.

But let me know that you are a brain injury survivor, and everything changes. I instantly know many of your deepest struggles, I know your pain, your sense of bewilderment, your sense of confusion, your anger and all else that can encompass life after a brain injury occurs.

In all probability, I understand a large part of you that remains a mystery to those closest to you – the uninjured souls who remain in your life. I liken it to meeting a close family member that you have not seen in a couple of years, simply picking things up where we left off last time.

I find this to be one of the silver linings in my own life as a brain injury survivor. Over the years, I have met hundreds who share my fate. Sometimes these meetings happen in unsurprising places – like brain injury conferences.

Meanwhile, at other times, these 'chance meetings' seem to come out of the blue, at the most unexpected times. It's the latter that I love, those unpredicted passing of paths of two souls that seem to come purely by chance, leaving you wondering if there really is something mysterious guiding us as we meander through life.

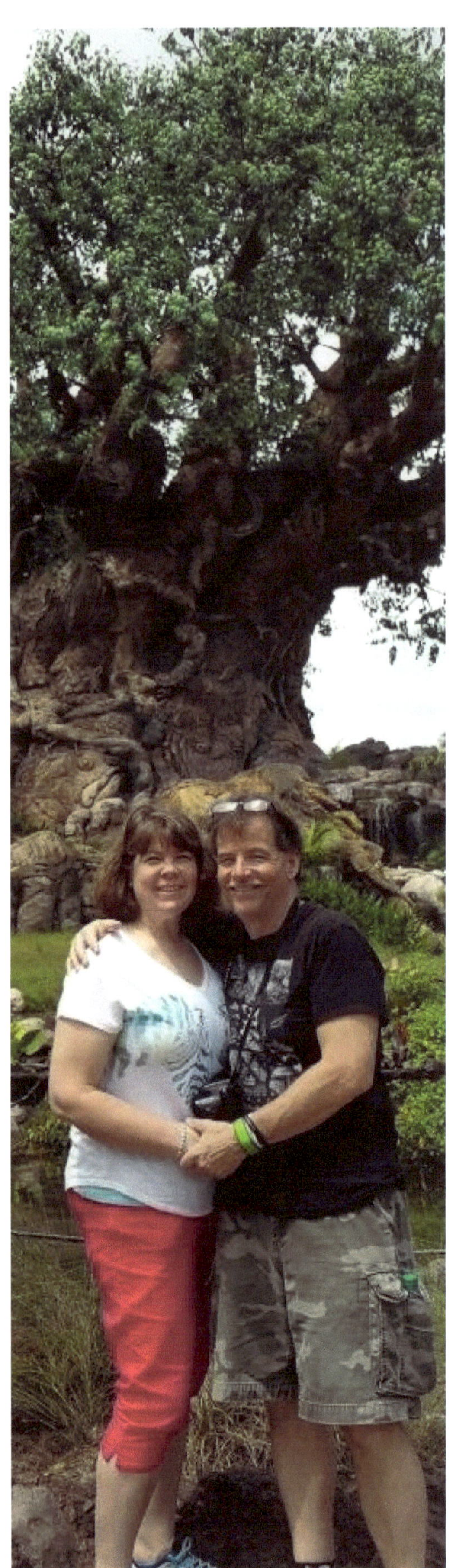

And so it came to pass on a recent conversation with a Disney cast member.

Sarah and I have long been fans of All Things Disney. Before life changed rather abruptly back in 2010, it wasn't uncommon for the two of us to travel from New Hampshire to Walt Disney World several times a year. We are both a couple of big kids on the inside, so our love for Disney wasn't a surprise to anyone who knew us.

There was never any arrogance about our frequent trips south. On virtually every trip we would pause for a moment, perhaps on Main Street, USA, or at times in Future World in Epcot, and say the same thing, "There are people making a once-in-a-lifetime trip here today." We would again share quietly with each other how blessed we were. We took nothing for granted.

Then, catastrophe struck in the form of a teenage driver plowing me down while I cycled. Lots of life has happened in the seven years since that not-so-wonderful day. But against odds higher than Space Mountain, we rebuilt our lives.

We no longer travel with the frequency that we did in our lives before the accident. PTSD and a dramatic elimination of my ability to work meant that life was downsized significantly. When you have less, you do less. We did less, focusing for years on doing things together that were free (or close to it), and that did not involve being around crowds. PTSD does have a way of making a small, more intimate life look much more attractive.

Last year was a breakthrough year in my recovery. Back to work full-time and reengaging in life feels a bit like being reborn. Whoever thought that my seventh year would be my best year? Ever so slowly, Sarah and I are reengaging in life. I will never say that I am fully recovered from my brain injury, but I am also not the person I was a few short years ago, and certainly not the same person I was during the first year or two after brain injury tried to darken our future and steal our hope.

Recently we made the decision to head back to our Happy Place. I have always been the family travel planner, almost obsessively looking for the best deals on flights, hotels, flights & hotels, and finding a way to travel as affordably as possible. Over the years I've learned that very careful trip planning saves a lot of money.

For reasons that are not that important to anyone but Sarah and me, I had to make a small change to our Disney hotel reservation. Unable to make the change online, I called Disney directly, knowing that cast members had access to options that were not on the Disney website.

It was there that my conversation with Devi started.

For those unaware of Disney policy, the names on cast member badges are not always the real names of those wearing them, and the same goes for cast members on the phone.

"I need to make a change to our upcoming reservation, Devi," I shared – always over excited speaking to anyone from Disney.

For the next fifteen minutes, we chit-chatted as she attempted to work a bit of magic that would allow us to stay in one hotel, rather than splitting our stay over two locations. She was adept at multitasking and I heard her fingers flying on her keyboard at the same time we exchanged pleasantries. While I am always courteous, I go out of my way to be a bit extra-nice when I am speaking with anyone who works with the public. Not everyone shares my attitude, so I know that it makes life a bit easier for some, albeit for a short while.

> "These days I am less apt to use the term traumatic brain injury than I did early on."

Devi knew we were Disney regulars already, our past trips forever stamped in the WDW database. "We slowed our trips down a few years ago as I was recovering from an accident."

"What happened, if you don't mind me asking," Devi asked with sincere interest.

Where would I even begin to start on an open-ended question like that? These days I am less apt to use the term traumatic brain injury than I did early on, but for whatever reason, on that day, at that time, on that call, I did. I shared the very short version – I was hit, life sucked big-time, years passed, and things are okay now for the first time in a long time.

End of story – or so I thought.

"David, I had a brain injury a few years ago. I hit my head on concrete coming out of a tunnel at an aquarium. It took a long time for me to be diagnosed with a brain injury."

At that instant, the conversation changed abruptly. I was no longer just a guest calling in; we were immediately part of the same extended family. For the next few minutes, we shared stories, anecdotes, and tales common to those of us within the brain injury community. Like her, I was back to work. I commented on her ability to multitask, solving complex problems with relative ease. She was clearly happy to be speaking with someone who understood how hard she had worked to get to this point.

As our call wound down, we parted as friends. She asked again about the name of our magazine, with the intent of subscribing. She may even read this article. Stranger things have happened. It's those chance meetings with others who share our fate, survivors like Devi Jolly, that make life interesting. And to know that others are able to slowly rebuild lives after brain injury still offers me so much hope, knowing that others have accomplished what I strive to.

These days, when life has us out and about, I occasionally wonder if someone we cross paths with is "in the club," but I never ask. Doing so is not really socially acceptable. But when the universe winks and someone shares their fate as a survivor, I just smile, both inside and out, knowing that we are everywhere.

Meet David A. Grant

David A. Grant is a freelance writer based out of southern New Hampshire as well as the founder and publisher of HOPE Magazine. He is the author of Metamorphosis, Surviving Brain Injury. He is also a contributing author to Chicken Soup for the Soul, Recovering from Traumatic Brain Injuries. David is a BIANH Board Member and a regular contributing writer to Brainline.org, a PBS sponsored website.

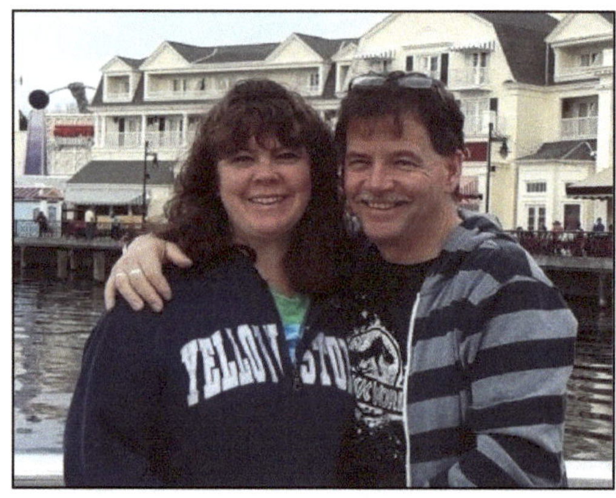

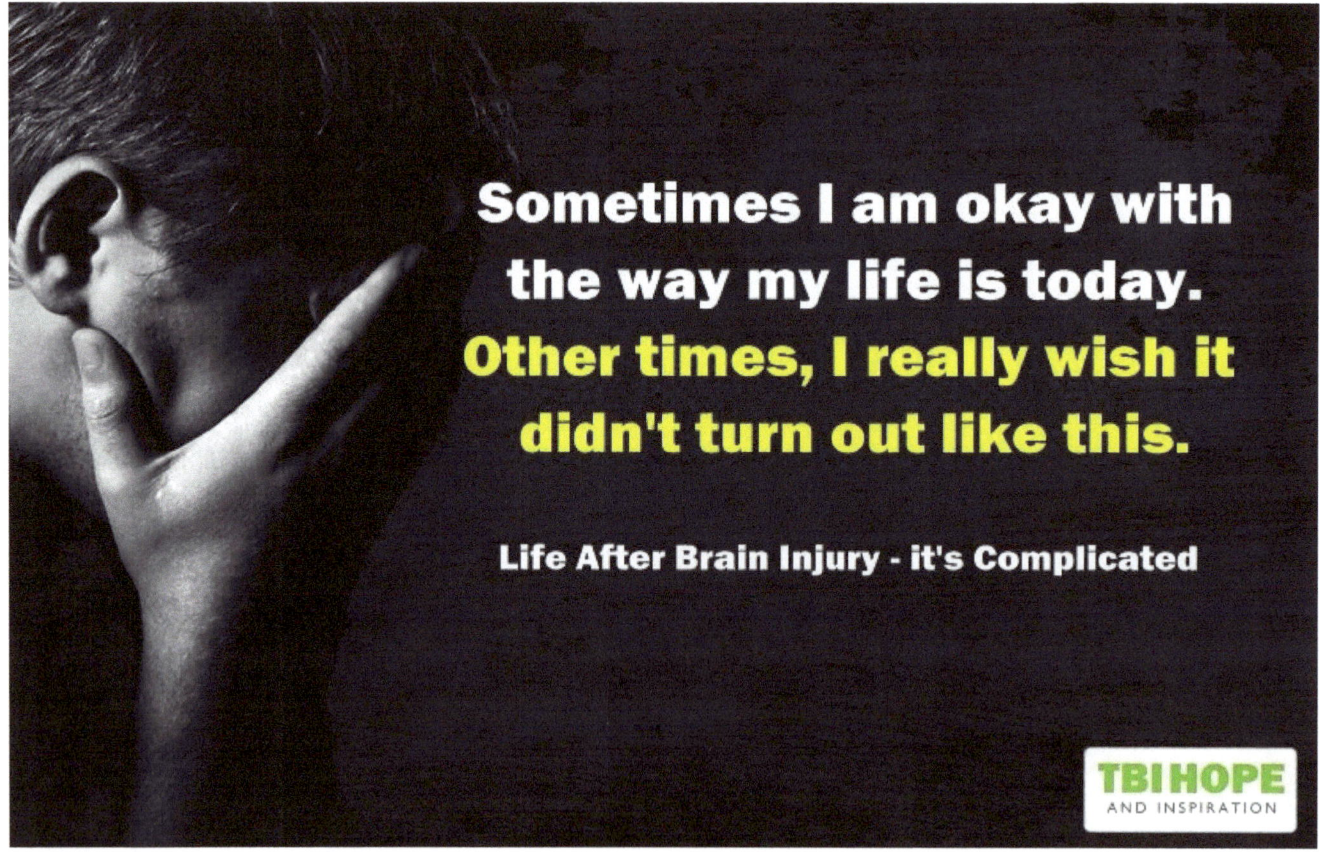

INTRODUCING THE NEW

dish FLEX PACK

Create Your Own TV Package

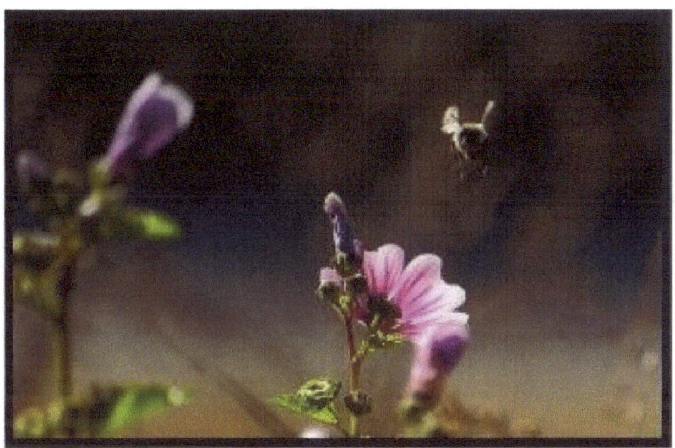

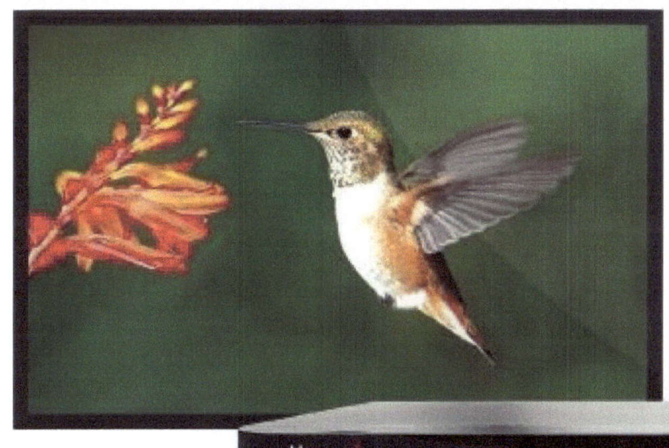

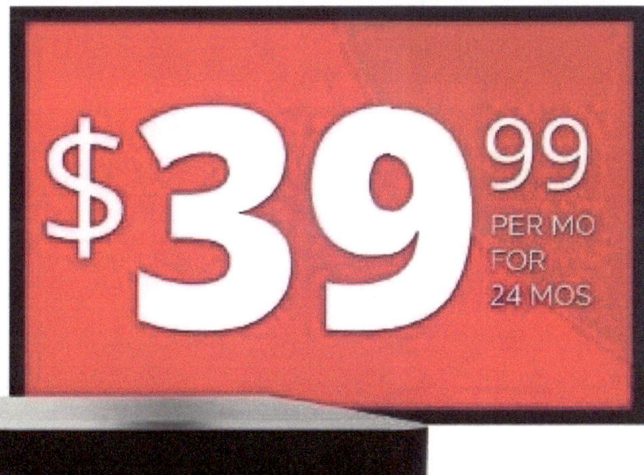

Free Streaming

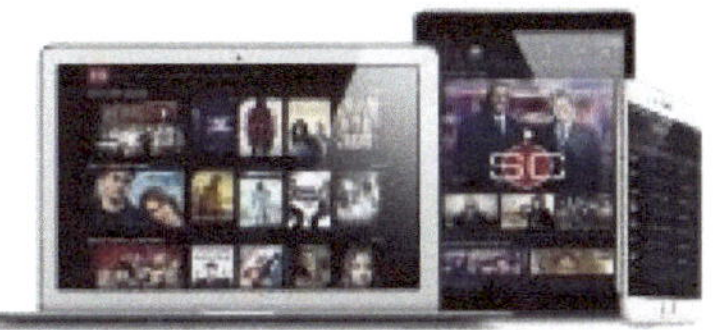

on all of your devices

Free Installation

\+

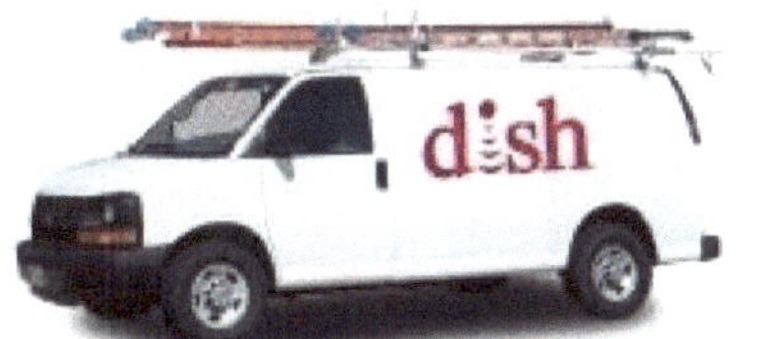

Add Internet

\+

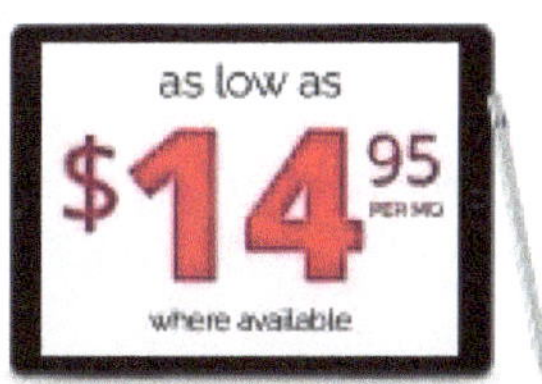

Call 1-800-391-1328

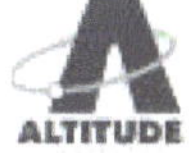

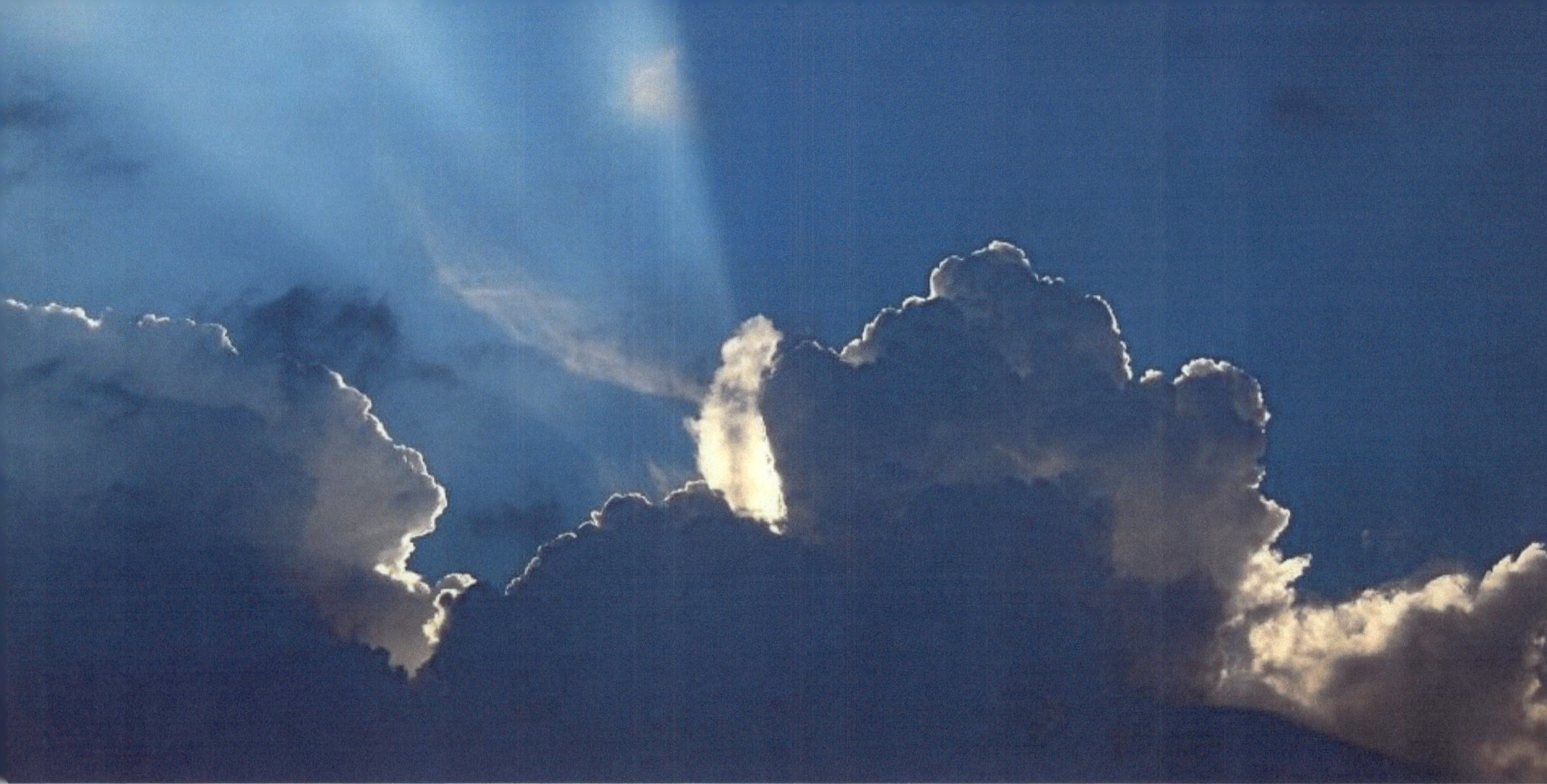

Silver Linings

By Norma Myers

If you mentioned the words *silver lining* to me in conjunction with the loss of our first-born son, Aaron, and our only surviving son, Steven, fighting for his life with a severe Traumatic Brain Injury (TBI) my *kind* response would have been, "*Are you absolutely crazy?*" When you open your door to police officers with pained faces that spoke before they could audibly voice the words of our sons being in a fatal accident, you can't fathom being able to breathe again, to experience happiness again, let alone think there could ever be silver linings after such a life-changing event.

The words *silver lining* did not appear in the unwelcomed TBI manual that was dutifully placed in my unsteady hands. I will never forget the feeling of that manual; it weighed as much as a magazine, yet felt like a cold cinderblock leaving me with an urge to thrust it out the ICU window. I felt like I needed an interpreter as my own traumatized brain attempted to decipher such words as Intracranial Pressure (ICP), Craniotomy, and neurostorming, just to name a few.

> You get the picture. These are words no parent should ever hear.

You get the picture. These are words no parent should ever hear.

In those early hours after attempting to absorb the shock, my head and heart kept screaming for me to go to Aaron. Even while drowning in his own pain, my husband repeatedly reminded me there was nothing we could do for Aaron. We both knew Aaron would expect us to run to Steven's rescue, just as he had done numerous times himself.

Despite being repeatedly told that Steven wouldn't make it, we did exactly what Aaron would do: we stood vigil over Steven's fragile, unrecognizable body. We prayed for his survival, not that he would be whole and perfect, because none of us are. We just needed our son to live. Deficits never entered our minds. We just needed him, as much as he needed us. The truth is, we needed him more. Which leads us to our first silver lining, Steven survived! Against all odds, he is our silver lining of *all* silver linings!

During Steven's many years of rehabilitation, when my physical, emotional and spiritual tanks ran empty, when exhaustion hit so hard that not even a double shot of espresso coupled with dark chocolate could revive me, silver linings showed up in the form of everyday people including:

- Doctors who offered hugs versus another dreaded diagnosis;
- Therapists who refused to give up;
- Nurses who cared for our son while taking extra time to care for his mom and dad;
- Family members, friends, community, good Samaritans and total strangers who put their lives on hold to come to our rescue.

All of these compassionate people shared our motto: "Whatever it takes!" These priceless gold nuggets showed up, illuminating the darkest of days, providing welcomed rays of hope.

"Despite being repeatedly told that Steven wouldn't make it, we did exactly what Aaron would do: we stood vigil over Steven's fragile, unrecognizable body."

My husband, Carlan, and I will never forget the moment when Steven turned the corner. It was none other than the day of Aaron's Life Celebration. *That's right!* We couldn't believe the timing either, but we indeed had two celebrations on that day. I often think Aaron planned it that way. He always wanted to be in the spotlight, but on this brotherly day, he insisted that the spotlight shine on Steven. Steven shone brightly, holding nothing back to make his big brother proud. He came back to us on Aaron's day. As brothers, best friends, how fitting that they shared the same day to celebrate two precious lives!

A silver lining that is near and dear to my heart is related to our marriage. According to our wise counselor, the chance for a marriage to survive trauma was not encouraging. There is no documented data, no statistic for marriages that survive double trauma. I thank God every day, that our marriage has withstood the test of all tests. Our vows, *for better, for worse, for richer, for poorer, in sickness and in health,* took on an entirely new and cherished meaning.

I can't end my blog without thanking Aaron for teaching us about the silver lining of being *noticers*. Being a person who notices nature and people—especially those that are hurting—was an example, a gift that Aaron passed down to Steven. I often think of how Aaron wanted to rescue everyone. He took time to be present.

To listen. To hug, real tight. To smile while offering words of assurance that regardless of present circumstances, everything will be okay if you don't give up. He believed those words and lived them with his whole heart, and we see Steven doing the same.

At the end of each day, we all have choices. We can be bitter, angry, isolate or get mad at God—all of which I have experienced. These choices left me empty, unfulfilled, and confused. I'm thankful that I didn't lose myself in empty choices. Instead, while living with a permanently scarred heart from the earthly loss of Aaron, I attempt to focus on basking in the glow of silver linings; to remain thankful for the blessings right in front of me; to be present for those that love and need me.

Meet Norma Myers

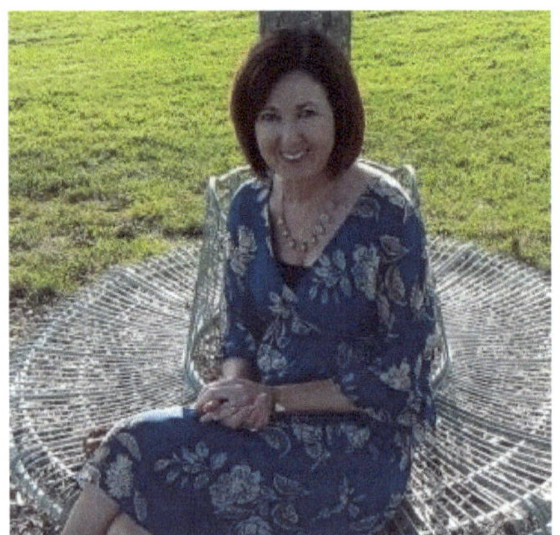

Norma and her husband Carlan spend much of their time supporting their son Steven as he continues on his road to recovery. Norma is an advocate for those recovering from traumatic brain injury.

Her written work has been featured on Brainline.org, a multi-media website that serves the brain injury community. Her family continues to heal.

News & Views

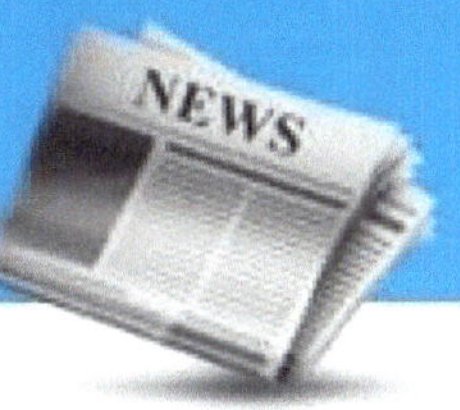

You have just read our thirty-sixth issue of HOPE Magazine. The stories shared in this month's issue are among some of the most powerful stories we have published. A mother's love for one son lost, and another forever changed. The passing of a beloved husband due at least in part to challenges with a brain

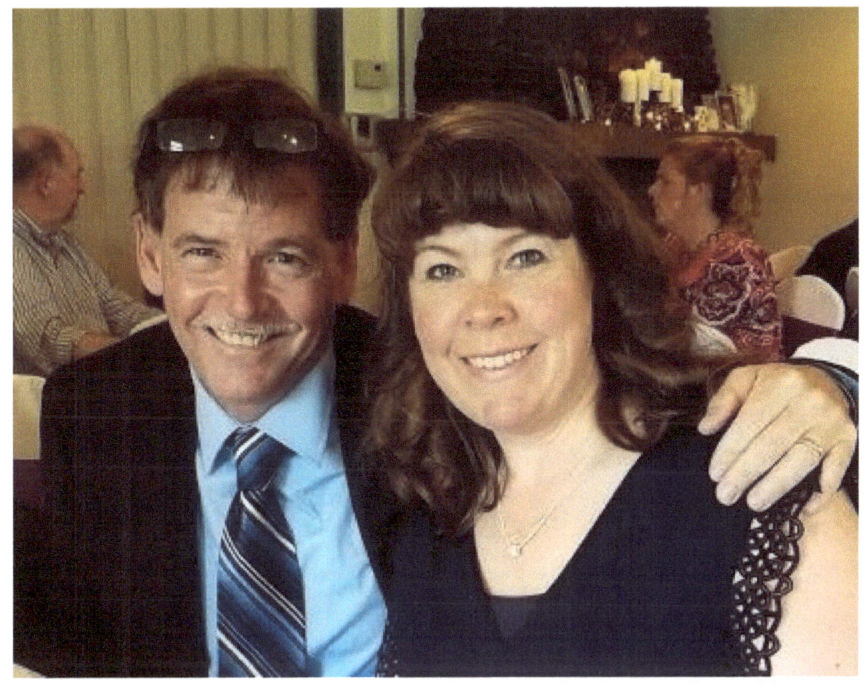

injury he sustained years ago, a mom who delights in helping her son enjoy life to the best of his ability as a brain injury survivor. Then there are the stories by survivors themselves, most all beating the odds and finding a way to live meaningful lives.

Though I try to maintain as much objectivity as possible, this issue moved me deeply, several times to tears, as I worked through the magazine layout.

Brain injury is such a complicated thing to try to describe – and even more complicated to live with. I know this from living as a survivor. But the stories in this issue shine a light on the humanity of brain injury, the kindness of souls who do all they can to support others, and simply amazing courage shown by those willing to share the toughest chapters of their lives. They have my utmost respect and admiration.

I encourage you to be kind, to extend a helping hand wherever you can, and to perhaps reflect on the fact that together we can do what none of us is capable of doing alone.

We wish you well on your journey.

~David & Sarah